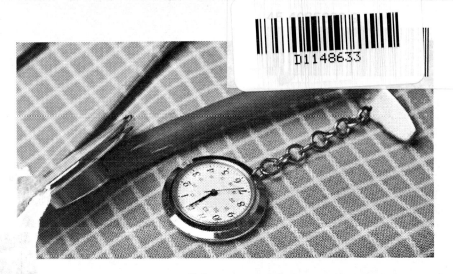

Succeeding in your Application to Nursing

How to prepare the perfect UCAS Personal Statement

Matt Green

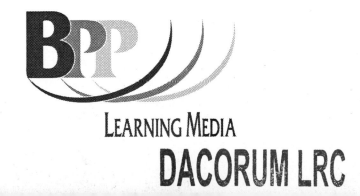

LEARNING MEDIA

DACORUM LRC

First edition September 2011

ISBN 9781 4453 7962 3

British Library Cataloguing-in-Publication Data
A catalogue record for this book is available from the British Library

Published by
BPP Learning Media Ltd
BPP House, Aldine Place
London W12 8AA

www.bpp.com/health

Typeset by Replika Press Pvt Ltd, India
Printed in the United Kingdom

The views expressed in this book are those of BPP Learning Media and not those of UCAS. BPP Learning Media are in no way associated with or endorsed by UCAS.

The contents of this book are intended as a guide and not professional advice. Although every effort has been made to ensure that the contents of this book are correct at the time of going to press, BPP Learning Media, the Editor and the Author make no warranty that the information in this book is accurate or complete and accept no liability for any loss or damage suffered by any person acting or refraining from acting as a result of the material in this book.

Every effort has been made to contact the copyright holders of any material reproduced within this publication. If any have been inadvertently overlooked, BPP Learning Media will be pleased to make the appropriate credits in any subsequent reprints or editions.

Contents

Contents

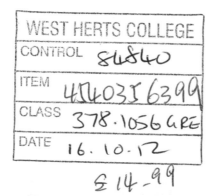

About the Publisher

BPP Learning Media is dedicated to supporting aspiring professionals with top quality learning material. BPP Learning Media's commitment to success is shown by our record of quality, innovation and market leadership in paper-based and e-learning materials. BPP Learning Media's study materials are written by professionally-qualified specialists who know from personal experience the importance of top quality materials for success.

About the Author

Matt Green BSc (Hons) MPhil

Matt Green has spent the last six years directly helping tens of thousands of individuals successfully apply to university. It is with this extensive experience in mind that Matt has written this book to help applicants prepare an effective UCAS Personal Statement as part of their application to university.

Acknowledgements

I would like to thank all of the prospective university students I have supported in the past six years; they have enabled the writing of this book to become a reality.

I would also like to thank my editor, Jen Morris, whose dedication has made this project possible.

Preface

This informative guide is intended to help applicants to universities in the United Kingdom submit an effective, compelling Personal Statement. It will assist school leavers, graduates and mature applicants alike, as well as parents and teachers. Please use this guide alongside advice provided by your school or college, from the Universities and College Admissions Service (UCAS), and assistance offered by the universities themselves.

This guide includes examples of 'Personal Statements' in order to illustrate certain key principles. It is vitally important that you see them as they are – illustrative examples.

The most important aspect of your Personal Statement is that it is written by, and is about, you!

Chapter 1

Applying to study Nursing in the United Kingdom: The process

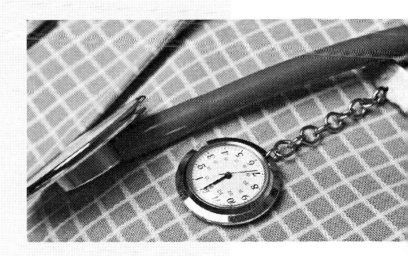

Applying to study Nursing in the United Kingdom: The process

In 2009 there were over 43,000 applications to pre-registration Nursing programmes in the United Kingdom. In 2010, entries to nursing programmes increased to just under 60,000 with under half of all applicants accepted.

As the competition for university places continues to increase, the need for a clear, engaging and well-structured application is paramount. It is with this in mind that we have produced this informative guide to help you succeed in your application to study Nursing.

With over six years experience of delivering bespoke help and support to prospective university students, we have amassed a wealth of insider insight into the university admissions process, and have distilled a winning formula for writing engaging and, most importantly, successful Personal Statments.

The UCAS application

All applications to universities in the United Kingdom are made through the Universities and Colleges Admission Service (UCAS). If you are at school or college, the application process will be co-ordinated by the head of post-16 education and you will be provided with login details and instructions on how to proceed. If you are applying as a graduate or mature student not currently in full time education, you can register with UCAS directly in order to submit your application.

Prospective students must submit their university applications via UCAS using the somewhat daunting 'UCAS application form' which is now in electronic format. Although the paper based 'UCAS form' is not commonly used now for applications to university, the electronic application process still requires all the information that would have been previously submitted. Accordingly, the electronic UCAS form requires you to enter your personal details, your course choices, your predicted or actual grades, your reference and your Personal Statement.

When considering an application to university, the admissions tutors place particular emphasis upon your academic performance, your reference and your Personal Statement. Indeed, some universities currently make offers to students based solely on their applications without conducting any interviews.

The importance of your UCAS Personal Statement

Your university Personal Statement is hugely important, arguably **the** most important passage you will ever write about yourself. As more and more universities move away from routinely interviewing applicants, the Personal Statement section of the UCAS application represents your first and last chance to make a strong, lasting and positive impression on the admissions tutors. Bearing in mind that university is a place where many people really develop as individuals, experience new things and ultimately determine their future career, the importance of your UCAS Personal Statement should not be underestimated. However, nor should the prospect of writing it be one you should fear. Far from it – it should be viewed as your opportunity to tell the world exactly why you are a special person, and to convince your chosen universities that they would be foolish not to offer you a place to study on your chosen course.

The art of writing is in the expression of ideas or information in a contolled, well crafted but ultimately compelling fashion. The key to great writing is in the balance of content and form: a voluminous vocabulary and a poet's aptitude for eloquent expression are all well and good, but they can appear superficial in the absence of an interesting subject or supporting facts. Likewise, the most compelling idea or important information will lose all of its impact and interest if it is buried in reams of

3

clumsy, tedious and poorly constructed prose. Ensuring that the content and expression work together to impress the reader is a skill in itself. So how exactly does this little essay on the essence of fine writing relate to your UCAS Personal Statement?

Imagine the university selection process from the point of view of an admissions tutor. Picture your desk lost beneath a heap of innumerable Personal Statements: are you relishing the prospect of carefully reading through them all, pausing every now and then to marvel at the number of extra-curricular activities here, nodding in admiration at the achievement of a Gold Duke of Edinburgh Award there? If you have detected that this question carries with it a hint of cynicism, then we are sure you appreciate the point we are trying to make: admissions tutors read hundreds of Personal Statements each year, and so it is imperative that yours makes an immediate, lasting and obviously positive impact. In short, you need to 'stand out from the crowd'.

While it is true that you can do little to improve **what** you will say (short of participating in a few last-minute extra-curricular activites in a desperate bid to appear super keen), it is well within your power to vastly improve **how** you will say it. In business this is termed as 'selling yourself' but, to put a slightly less commercial spin on it, it is essentially all about giving the best possible account of yourself in order to move one step closer to realising the hopes and aspirations you hold for your future.

At present, the UCAS Personal Statement must be completed within 4,000 characters. It is also important to note that when entering the Personal Statement onto the UCAS system, any formatting – such as underlining, italics or bolding – will be lost.

So, **your** UCAS Personal Statement is **your** key opportunity to convince university admissions tutors that **you** are an exceptional candidate and that they should offer **you** a place at their university over other applicants. It is vital that you make your comments clearly and compellingly, so that the admissions tutors become really keen to meet you and find out more about the special, unique person that you are!

How a UCAS Personal Statement enhances your university application

In terms of how your university application will be assessed, there are four crucially important strands:

- Your predicted grades
- Your employment history (more important for mature applicants)
- Your character reference
- Your Personal Statement

Although you have some degree of control over the person you choose to provide a reference for you, by the time you come to put together your application form, your predicted grades and reference lie largely outside of your control. The only aspect of your application over which you have complete control is your Personal Statement. Another factor to consider is that, even if you have been predicted three As at A level, given the growing popularity of Nursing courses, many of your fellow applicants will have similarly impressive predicted grades. In this situation, it will be the Personal Statement which will be used as the chief criteria on which judgements over acceptance or rejection are based. Similarly, supposing that your reference is full of glowing praise – so will those of the vast majority of other applicants, because if anyone needs a reference, it is common sense that they will ask people who they anticipate will speak highly of them. So, having established that great predicted grades and a glowing reference are par for the course in the world of university applications, we are left with the conclusion that the most important aspect of your university application is your Personal Statement.

Chapter 1

Ultimately, a Personal Statement represents your opportunity to introduce yourself to the admissions tutors in order to give them a clear idea of you as a person, along with what makes you 'tick'.

Key points

Make sure that you first make contact with UCAS and the universities themselves in order to find out *exactly* what you need to do when applying to study Nursing.

Attending university Open Days is especially valuable; you have the chance then to ask questions directly.

Remember, whilst your grades and reference are equally important, your Personal Statement is the only element of your UCAS application that is completely within your control.

Chapter 2

What kind of students do Nursing tutors want?

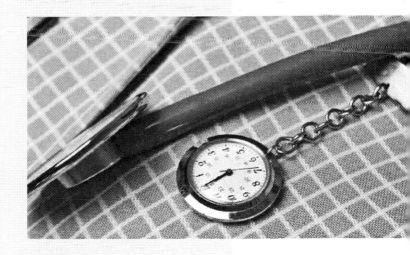

What kind of students do Nursing tutors want?

Through our experience supporting individuals in their applications to study Nursing, we have formed a solid understanding of the guiding principles used by universities in the selection and admission of students.

These are:

1. **Selection for a Nursing degree implies selection for the nursing profession**
    A degree in Nursing confirms academic achievement and in normal circumstances entitles the new graduate to be provisionally registered with the Nursing and Midwifery Council (NMC).
2. The selection process attempts to identify the core academic and non-academic qualities of a nurse:
    *   **Honesty, integrity** and an ability to **recognise one's own limitations** and those of others, are central to the practice of nursing.
    *   Other key attributes include having **good communication** and **listening skills**, an ability **to make decisions under pressure**, and to **remain calm and cope with stress.**
    *   Nurses must have an understanding of **teamwork** and respect for the contributions of others. Desirable characteristics include **compassion, initiative, flexibility and integrity.**
3. A high level of academic attainment will be expected. A good understanding of the Sciences is key to Nursing but universities genrally encourage diversity in subjects studied by candidates.
4. The practice of nursing requires the highest standards of **professional** and **personal conduct**. Put simply, some students will not be suited to a career in nursing and it

is in the interests of the student and the public that they should not be admitted to university.

5.   The practice of nursing requires the highest standards of **professional competence**. However, a history of serious ill health or disability will not jeopardise a career in nursing unless the condition impinges upon professional fitness to practise.

6.   Candidates should demonstrate some understanding of what a career in nursing involves and their suitability for a caring profession. Universities expect candidates to have had some relevant experience in a healthcare or related setting.

7.   The **primary duty of care is to patients.** All applicants to Nursing degrees will be expected to understand the importance of this principle.

8.   Failure to declare information that has a material influence on a student's fitness to practise may lead to termination of their Nursing course.

Clearly, it is important that you consult the websites of the universities to which you intend to apply in order to learn of any specific requirements they are seeking.

University education is also expensive. For every student who drops out, there are financial implications to the university. **So, one of the most important questions to be considered in the admissions process is: will the student complete the course?**

Finally, universities are also looking for students who will contribute to the broad spectrum of university life. Those who do so are so much more likely to gain a wider experience of working and communicating with people from different backgrounds.

The admissions tutor's perspective

In deciding who will and who will not to be invited to study Nursing at their institution, universities look to the views of their admissions tutors, the people who read the application submissions and who conduct the interviews.

And when reading hundreds of Personal Statements, so often the key considerations of the tutors are:

'Does this candidate have a sense of what they are going to get into by studying Nursing, and indeed by studying Nursing at this university?'

'Can I see this individual becoming a good practicing nurse in a few years from now?'

Whilst it is likely that admissions tutors will be looking to see if you possess the personal qualities so often associated with nurses – qualities such as kindness, compassion, empathy, and curiosity – they are perhaps even more determined to see if you are always reliable, and that you can handle the physical, mental and emotional strains you will experience, firstly as a student and, eventually, as a professional nurse.

Key points

Selection for a Nursing degree implies selection for the nursing profession.

Universities want candidates with more than academic ability. They want to train the nurses of tomorrow.

Chapter 3

The essential contents of the Personal Statement

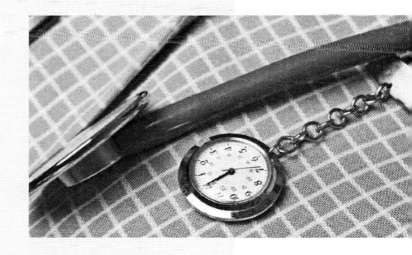

The essential contents of the Personal Statement

Your Personal Statement is your opportunity to describe in words:

a. The reasons why you are so keen to study Nursing, and at the universities to which you are submitting your applications.
b. That even in advance of taking up your nursing studies, you have already made a real commitment to this course of action by gaining relevant experience.
c. That you have a good idea of, and are equipped to handle, the expectations, responsibilities, pressures and duties attached to the practice of nursing.
d. That you are special, and possess attributes which will see you through your Nursing course and towards establishing your professional career.

Let us take each of these themes above and look at them carefully.

What is Nursing?

> 'Nursing is an applied vocational and academic discipline practised in a variety of complex situations. Nursing focuses on promoting health and helping individuals, families and groups to meet their health care needs. The work involves assisting people whose autonomy is impaired and who may present a range of disabilities or health related problems. Nurses work with patients, clients, families and communities in primary care, acute and critical care, rehabilitation and tertiary care settings.
>
> UCAS website July 2010

Pre-registration Nursing programmes

All approved pre-registration courses in the United Kingdom lead to registration with the Nursing and Midwifery Council (NMC). Currently, applicants can choose one of two options available for pre-registration training; degree based programmes (BSc Hons) or diploma courses (Dip HE).

However, all Nursing courses commencing from September 2013 will be degree based only. Universities offering diploma courses will be phasing these out between September 2011 and early 2013. It is vital that you contact individual institutions close to the time of your application to find out where they are in the process and what options are available to you.

There is very little difference between pre-registration degree and diploma courses. However, in order to be selected for degree level, applicants are usually required to have a higher standard of academic achievement and will subsequently undertake a more academically intense programme. Subjects receiving more attention in degree based study include biology, sociology, psychology and physiology. Course content and entry requirements will vary between institutions and you should refer to individual university websites in order to gain a full understanding of the programmes to which you are applying.

Both degree and diploma courses consist of 50% theory and 50% practice, with time divided between university based study and practical experience with approved placement providers. Students usually take a common foundation programme in the first year before specialising in one of four branches; Learning Disability Nursing, Children's Nursing (Paediatrics), Mental Health Nursing or Adult Nursing.

Learning Disability Nursing

Learning Disability Nurses work with vulnerable members of society, their families and their carers to ensure an optimum standard of living and, as a result, optimum health. Care is usually provided within community based or residential settings.

The primary focus of Learning Disability Nursing is to provide individualised care plans for clients, allowing them to live their lives as fully and independently as possible. Attention is paid to basic life and social skills and to integrating individuals into an inclusive society irrespective of disability.

Children's Nursing (Paediatrics)

Paediatric Nurses provide appropriate care to children and young people suffering from a wide range of conditions. It is imperative that those working in Children's Nursing have an in-depth knowledge of the requirements of young people and how these change during the different stages of development.

Paediatric care takes place within a range of settings, including hospitals and homes, as well as in the community.

Mental Health Nursing

Mental Health Nurses work with individuals of all ages who suffer from a range of mental health problems. The focus is on a client based approach, providing individualised care to aid patients in their recovery, or in learning to adjust to life dealing with mental health problems.

Nurses working in mental health do so in a variety of capacities. These include community and residential settings as well as working within the NHS or private hospitals and secure units.

Adult Nursing

A wide variety of roles exist under the umbrella of Adult Nursing, but the main focus lies in providing care and support to individuals suffering or recovering from illness and disease.

Mainly based in hospitals or the community, Adult Nurses may be involved in caring for patients with chronic diseases such as diabetes, serious acute conditions such as strokes, preparing patients for surgery, assisting those admitted to accident and emergency or in need of tests and assessments.

By all means, use your Personal Statement to demonstrate where your specific nursing career interests presently lie **but** also understand that your views may well change in the light of your education and practical experiences.

What the universities say

In order to gear your Personal Statement in the right direction, it can be highly useful to consult individual university websites and consider their definition of the nursing profession and the qualities and attributes required to be successful in it.

Presented below are a series of statements from a small selection of universities for you to consider. Ideally, to gain a full understanding of each course and its requirements, applicants should refer the websites of each institution to which they are applying.

> *'The focus of attention for a nurse is the patient, not simply the condition, but the needs and anxieties which it may generate, including pressures on family and friends. The mark of a professional nurse is the ability to observe and assess what is happening to a patient and to select the most effective response.'*

> *'Nursing also requires intellectual capacity, coupled with a genuine desire to care for others. Nursing is all about caring for people, and delivering that care demands exceptional skills of exceptional people.'*
> Buckinghamshire New University website July 2010

'To become a nurse you need to be people-focused, have excellent communication skills, and a caring approach to your work. You must have dedication, passion and a commitment to delivering high quality healthcare to those who need it.'

City University website July 2010

'Nurses are in a unique position within the health care provision, and can work in a wide variety of settings. It involves caring for individuals, families and communities in order to maintain levels of good health. It can be a demanding career, but can also be incredibly fulfilling and rewarding, and it can provide you with a choice of career pathways which can change over the years.'

De Montfort University website July 2010

'As a qualified nurse you will care for, support and educate people of all ages. Once qualified, many nurses take extra courses to specialise in areas such as cancer care, women's health, accident and emergency, critical care, practice nursing, health visiting or school nursing.

'Nursing can also encompass a wide range of activities depending on your career choice. It's not just about caring for people who are unwell; it can also include promoting health, educating, advising or using your skills and knowledge in management or specialist roles.'

University of Chester website July 2010

The quotations above deserve careful consideration when compiling your Personal Statement. Not only do they give an overview of the nursing profession, they provide a solid starting point from which to begin drafting out your ideas.

For example, look at the ways in which a career in nursing is described: in particular, note the use of words such as *'fulfilling'*, *'demanding'* and *'rewarding'*.

Look also at the personal attributes required of healthcare professionals. For example, *'dedication, passion and a commitment to delivering high quality healthcare'* and *'intellectual capacity, coupled with a genuine desire to care for others'*.

When writing your Personal Statement, you must write it in your own words and style. However, admissions tutors will be looking for evidence of **enthusiasm** and careful **reflection** in your comments. Be sure to demonstrate your understanding of nursing as a career, the challenges posed by studying the subject at university, and the personal qualities that make you a suitable candidate for your chosen course.

Why Nursing at this university?

Before you begin to write your Personal Statement you need to decide the university to which you wish to apply. It is important that you consult a careers advisor and visit the universities yourself before making your final decision. This is a decision not to be taken lightly given the fact that you will be dedicating the next several years to studying there.

There are many factors to take into account when considering your choice, including:

- Would you prefer to study at a campus or city-based university?
- Do you feel comfortable in the locality in which the university is set?
- Will you get the opportunity to undertake research as part of the course?
- When would you start interacting with patients?
- What extracurricular activities are available?
- Do you want to study close to your family home, or not?

Each university has a slightly different selection process so it is important that you also visit their website in order to obtain the necessary details.

Your commitment to Nursing studies and a nursing career

Consider the situation in which a Premier League football club is deliberating whether or not to offer a teenage boy, with aspirations to be a professional footballer, a position within the club's youth academy. You can be sure that in addition to their consideration of his football ability, the club's coaches will also be looking to see signs of a real commitment to a future career in the sport as demonstrated by, for example, his approach to diet, and his attitude to drinking and smoking. In short, the club will be keen to see evidence of personal investment in this career move. What is he keen to do; what is he prepared to give up?

The same applies in the consideration of university applications. The admissions tutors will be keen to find out how you spend your time outside the formal school curriculum.

For example, they may look to see if your Personal Statement contains evidence that:

- You try to keep abreast of relevant developments as they are reported in leading nursing journals (for example, *Nursing Standard*, *The BJN*) and the national newspapers, or
- You spend time at weekends supporting staff in a local hospice, care home or hospital.

Understanding the expectations, responsibilities and duties attached to the practice of nursing

The most authoritative description of the responsibilities and duties of nurses working in the United Kingdom is that issued by the Nursing and Midwifery Council (NMC), the body with which all nurses in the UK must become registered.

Presented below is an overview of the core principles of practice laid out by the NMC in 'The Code: Standards of conduct, performance and ethics for nurses and midwives'. **It is imperative that all applicants to Nursing degrees gain a full understanding of the NMC's requirements.**

The duties of a nurse registered with the NMC

Make the care of people your first concern, treating them as individuals and respecting their dignity:

- *Adopt a polite and compassionate approach toward patient care; respect the rights and beliefs of each individual and do not discriminate.*
- *Only use patient information for the purpose for which it was given and adopt responsibility for preventing any unauthorised access.*
- *Work collaboratively with those in your care, supporting and promoting personal wellbeing and healthcare.*
- *Gain consent before taking any action with regards to treatment and respect the patient's right to seek further consultation.*
- *Maintain professional boundaries at all times.*

Work with others to protect and promote the health and wellbeing of those in your care, their families and carers, and the wider community:

- *Work effectively as part of a team, sharing knowledge and skills where necessary, to ensure the best possible standards of patient care.*
- *Treat all colleagues with respect; do not discriminate.*

Provide a high standard of practice and care at all times:

- *Work within the confines of your skills and follow up to date guidelines for best practice in your relevant field.*
- *Recognise that you are responsible for continued professional development through lifelong learning; continually assess and update your knowledge and performance.*

Be open and honest, act with integrity and uphold the reputation of your profession:

- *Maintain the trust of the public, your patients and your colleagues through open, honest and professional behaviour.*
- *Understand and adhere to relevant regulations affecting both your work and your working environment.*
- *Recognise that you are responsible for upholding confidence, not only in yourself as a healthcare professional, but in the healthcare system as a whole.*

Accordingly, by drawing upon your experiences in life, especially your work experience, it is vital that you use your Personal Statement to convince the admissions tutors that you are able to:

- Engage appropriately with ill or disabled people, and
- Listen to them and support them, and
- Work effectively as a member of a team.

It is also important that you indicate your understanding of the physical and emotional demands placed upon nursing students and healthcare professionals.

As stated, the above is merely an overview of the responsibilties of a nurse working in the United Kingdom. For an in-depth description you should refer to material published by the NMC. Alongside the guiding principles for registered nurses, the NMC also sets out the responsibilities specific to students undertaking pre-registration training. These should be referred to when compiling ideas for your Personal Statement.

Show them you are special

When considering the Personal Statements of applicants to university, the admissions tutors will also be asking themselves:

- *Has this applicant really thought things through?*
- *Do we want to meet this candidate at interview?*
- *Do we see them enjoying and completing their studies, well on their way to becoming a good nurse?*
- *Will it be good for the university to have this candidate around?*

Your Personal Statement is your opportunity to influence the tutors towards saying 'Yes' in response to each of these questions as they apply to you!

So, it is important that you write in a way that depicts the enthusiasm, keenness – and indeed, **passion** – you have for your chosen academic choice.

Phrases such as 'I am *quite* interested in studying Nursing' or 'I really *think* that Nursing is the right course for me' are to be avoided; they are so unconvincing! And if you have received special commendations or prizes, write about them in a way that shows how they reinforce your decision to study Nursing.

For example, if you became Head Pupil at your school, this clearly shows the strength of the teachers' regard for your leadership qualities, and your ability to act as a role model for other pupils. So, elaborate upon those themes. Equally, if you worked effectively as part of a team raising money for your school's charity, you could describe how this experience improved your teamwork and communication skills.

It is vitally important when referring to your experiences in your Personal Statement to clearly state how these have developed in you the qualities that are required of a Nursing student and future nurse.

However, before you submit your final statement, you would also do well to talk about your 'special' qualities with your referee. Some comments are simply more effectively made by another person and it is important that your reference fully supports your application to university.

Key point

It is vital that you use your Personal Statement to convince the admissions tutors that you have really considered the implications of studying Nursing **and** that you know that it is right for you.

Chapter 4

Nursing applications: The myths

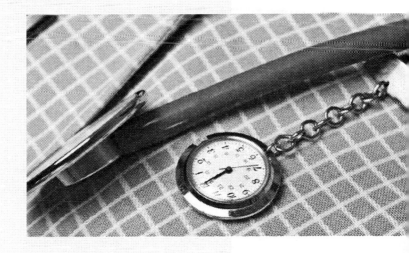

Nursing applications: The myths

During our experience in supporting students in their applications to study Nursing, we have come across many misunderstandings. Here are some which arise time after time:

1. **Universities are keen to meet students whose key motivation for wishing to become a nurse is due to a parent being a nurse.**
    No. Clearly, the fact that one of your parents is a nurse may very significantly account for your keen interest in studying Nursing. However, this is simply not sufficient justification for your decision to embark upon a career in the field. Admissions tutors will be looking to see how you have carefully considered your career options, and how you have confirmed your final choice by gaining appropriate experience.

2. **It is easier to gain admission to a pre-registration Nursing course if your parent is a nurse.**
    This is not true. Again, if your parent is a nurse it is certainly easier to gain an insight into the world of nursing. However, universities are interested in each individual applicant and in the steps they have undertaken to confirm that they have the right qualities for a future nursing career.

3. **Despite my greatest efforts I have been unable to secure work experience in a nursing environment therefore I will not be successful in my application to study Nursing.**
    Although for some people it may be difficult to secure work experience within a recognised nursing environment, there are many other options open to you that will enable you to gain first hand experience of working with ill, disabled or vulnerable people. Volunteering with organisations such as St John Ambulance or the Samaritans, or becoming involved with support groups for vulnerable clients, such as young offenders or people with disabilities, all offer the

chance for you to demonstrate relevant and transferable skills.

Remember, your work experience is crucial in enabling you to obtain first hand experience of working with, and helping to improve the quality of life of ill or disabled people, and confirming that you have what it takes to follow this through and establish a nursing career.

4. **As a male applicant my chances of gaining admission to a Nursing course are greatly reduced.**
This is simply not true. Indeed, there are a greater number of women than men working within the nursing profession however the number of male nurses is on the rise. Admissions tutors are interested in applicants who demonstrate dedication and commitment to a career in nursing, regardless of gender.

5. **When describing your work experience you should not refer to non-clinical experience.**
It can be extremely helpful to refer to your non-clinical experiences so long as you can justify how these have helped to equip you for your forthcoming studies, and beyond. For example, someone describing that they had led a mountaineering expedition would clearly demonstrate their strong leadership and teamwork skills.

6. **My Personal Statement must be exactly 4,000 characters or I will be penalised.**
Obviously, the more relevant information you include within the allowed space then the more fully you will be able to tell the admissions tutors about yourself and why you should be offered a place at their university. However, it really is about quality not quantity, so do not attempt to pad out your Personal Statement with irrelevant facts that do not add any value to your application or, worse still, weaken it.

7.   **Achieving good results in my examinations is the only thing I need to do to gain a place on a Nursing course.**
Not true at all. Yes, successful applicants to Nursing courses will obtain good academic results; however, it is vital that they also demonstrate that they have the qualities required of a good nurse. Think back to your own experiences when you may have been treated by a nurse: what special qualities made them stand out? Some of these include:

- Having a real desire to help people.
- Being able to communicate clearly.
- Understanding the importance of effective team working skills.
- Being empathic and honest.
- Recognising the importance of adopting a conscientious and highly motivated approach.

8.   **The sooner I submit my Personal Statement before the deadline the better my chances of success.**
This is another common misconception. The only real advantage of submitting your application as early as possible is that it will reduce your stress levels and enable you to concentrate on your studies. Despite what is commonly perceived, submitting your application earlier rather than later will not mean that you stand a better chance of your application progressing simply because it is at the top of the admission tutor's pile!

9.   **If I apply for a combination of degree and diploma programmes I will reduce my chances of admission.**
Admissions tutors will not think you are less committed to a particular entry route if you apply for a combination of degree and diploma courses. Indeed, unless the courses you have selected are at the same university, the Data Protection Act precludes admissions tutors the ability to identify your other applications.

Key point

Your Personal Statement is your opportunity to justify to the admissions tutors why **you**, as a **unique individual**, should be accepted on to a Nursing programme in the first step of a nursing career.

Chapter 5

Preparing your Personal Statement

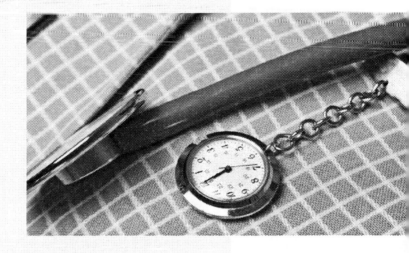

Preparing your Personal Statement

Check the key questions

The first step in preparing your Personal Statement is to take a good look at yourself – your personality, your strengths and your achievements. Then take a blank piece of paper and write down where you stand with regard to the key questions set out below. It is almost certain that you will not be able to touch upon each and every topic covered by these questions in your final Personal Statement. However, it will be helpful for you to consider each question; you can then decide which areas you are keen to include and which ones you are content to discard.

You might also find it valuable to have to hand the following when considering the key questions below:

- The list of the duties of a nurse registered with the NMC (page 19)
- The guiding principles adopted in the selection and admission of students to Nursing programmes (page 8)
- The definitions of nursing from university websites (pages 15–16)

But please note: it is extremely important that when it comes to writing your Personal Statement, you create your own expressions and phrases. Your Personal Statement has to be written uniquely in your style – about you!

Key questions

- When and why did you begin to be interested in nursing?
- Why do you want to study Nursing? Are you sure you want to be a nurse? Why do you want to be a nurse rather than, for example, a midwife, or an occupational therapist? Or a teacher?

- Why are you so keen to study Nursing at this particular university?
- What kind of person are you? Which aspects of your personality equip you well for the study of, and a subsequent career in, Nursing?
- What are your strengths and weaknesses? What are your strengths and weaknesses according to others, such as your parents, your friends, your teachers? What special talents do you have which could be of real value within a nursing career?
- What work experience have you had which has given you a special insight into life as a nursing student or as a nurse?
- What else have you done, or has happened to you, which has provided excellent learning experiences or drawn upon your special personal qualities, such as compassion, tenacity and empathy?
- What awards or prizes (academic and non-academic) have you received? What do these tell people about you?
- What are your keen interests outside academic studies?
- What do you see yourself doing in five or ten years' time?

Drafting a structure

When complete, an effective Personal Statement will comprise **three key sections**: your 'introduction', a 'conclusion', and between these two sections will lie those paragraphs comprising the 'main body' of the Personal Statement.

It is helpful to sketch onto a piece of blank paper three boxes; one labelled 'Introduction', one labelled 'Conclusion' and, lying between those two boxes, one labelled 'Main body'.

Now start mapping some draft comments to each of the three sections.

The introduction

The aim of the introduction is to catch the attention of the reader, namely the admissions tutor. So, try to compose a statement which really grabs the reader's attention and enables you to stand out from the crowd!

The main body of the Personal Statement

The main body of your Personal Statement is the section in which you build upon your introduction and describe:

- Why you have decided to study Nursing.
- The steps you have taken in making a real commitment to study Nursing.
- How you have a real sense of what studying Nursing, and a subsequent nursing career, entail.
- Aspects of yourself which especially equip you for this course of action.

It is in this section that you will refer to:

- Your work experience, and the relevant insights it has given you towards confirming that studying Nursing is right for you.
- The steps you have taken in furthering your interest in nursing and issues within the profession.
- The topics which you look forward to studying most.
- Your experience of teamwork, leadership and responsibility, reliability and tenacity.
- Your thoughts upon what direction your nursing career might take, always recognising that this might change in the light of experience at university.

The conclusion

It is vitally important to draw your Personal Statement to a close, and reaffirm that you are someone who will flourish academically and socially at university, and that you are well equipped to handle the stresses and strains associated with studying Nursing. The 'conclusion' paragraph is not the time to introduce any new themes. However, not to present a concise, summary comment would be a real error of judgement.

Writing and improving your Personal Statement

In formulating the contents of each of the key sections (introduction; main body; conclusion) of your Personal Statement, it is important that you focus upon the following questions:

- Do each of your sections, **especially the introduction,** and your Personal Statement as a whole have **real impact upon the reader?**
- Is the punctuation correct?
- Is the flow of your language appealing, non-repetitive and easy to follow?
- Is there a logical and coherent balance to the Personal Statement?
- Are all your statements absolutely honest and accurate? Remember! Anything you refer to in your Personal Statement may be the subject of questions at any subsequent interviews. Admissions tutors are very skilled at identifying situations where candidates have made exaggerated claims!
- Will the reader conclude that you are indeed 'special'? Is it truly about you?

And finally:

- **Have you concentrated on justifying and substantiating your comments?**

The admissions tutors will consider everything that you include in your Personal Statement to help them decide whether or not to offer you the opportunity to study Nursing at their university. It is not enough to write, for example: *'I want to study Nursing*

because Biology is my strongest subject, academically.' To excel in a specific academic subject is simply not sufficient justification for seeking to make a career within nursing and all that it entails.

Look again at this statement from a university from Chapter 3 and consider the qualities it lays out for a nurse:

> *'To become a nurse you need to be people-focused, have excellent communication skills, and a caring approach to your work. You must have dedication, passion and a commitment to delivering high quality healthcare to those who need it.'*

It clearly demonstrates that the nursing profession is as much about your personal attributes as it is your academic achievements.

You must maintain your own focus upon justifying and substantiating your comments throughout your entire Personal Statement.

Key points

You need time to write your Personal Statement, do not rush.

Prepare a first **draft**, containing an introduction, a main body and a conclusion.

Chapter 6

From 'Draft' to 'Refined': enhancing your Personal Statement

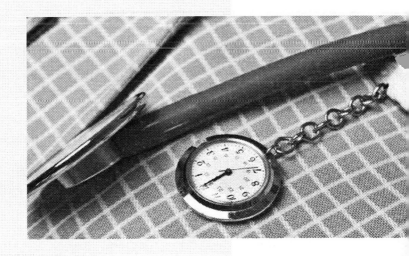

Chapter 6

From 'Draft' to 'Refined': enhancing your Personal Statement

One way in which we can illustrate the importance of focusing upon the key principles which govern the preparation of an effective, compelling Personal Statement is to consider a fictitious example, initially in its first 'draft' form, and then looking at it after some refinement. The critique which follows should not be interpreted as 'definitive', or 'state of the art'. And certainly, there is no such thing as the perfect Personal Statement. However, we hope that by using this scenario – moving from a 'draft' to a 'refined' version – we can bring the whole process to life!

Fictitious Personal Statement: 'Draft version'

I have always been interested in Adult Nursing so I would really like the chance to study this branch of nursing at university. Two members of my family are both respected nurses and my ambition is to hold a similarly rewarding position in the community.

I have thoroughly enjoyed studying A level in Biology and I also enjoy reading other books about developments in Science and I believe I will enjoy studying Nursing at university. To explore the subject further I have been to the Nurse Education Information Afternoon at York University in 2009.

I have also taken on some work experience in a range of nursing areas. I started in 2005 working at Hope House near Reading, which is a residential school for disabled children. I worked there every Wednesday and Saturday afternoon for two years during term-time. Last summer, I went with a group to Ireland for a week to work in a hospice as a volunteer looking after some of the patients there. This was a very demanding experience but it did not discourage me, rather it was one of the most amazing experiences of my life and I plan to return next year. I have also recently started a permanent position as a ward volunteer at Reading District General Hospital. I have also discussed

my future career with family members who work in nursing, and I am confident that I am well suited to this career.

I am a keen member of the school debating team and I am also captain of the hockey team, which has won several local tournaments. My involvement in the debating team has given me the chance to meet new people and develop skills in team working. Whilst playing in the hockey team has given me the chance to develop leadership skills and keep fit. I have also been involved in other extra-curricular activities through completing the Duke of Edinbourgh silver award. I am also a senior prefect. Art is another hobby of mine, and I like to visit various art galleries in my holidays. I love travelling and I have been to Canada, the USA, France, Italy and Spain. For this reason, I jumped at the chance of a gap year, and I will be working in Britain for six months before I set off travelling.

Character count: 2,145

Fictitious Personal Statement: 'Refined' version

Adult Nursing is a challenging and rewarding career that appeals to me as it combines my enjoyment of learning with my desire to contribute to improving people's health and wellbeing. As several of my relatives are nurses, I have benefited from discussions with them about the realities of a nursing career and about the need for communication skills and stamina in order to be a successful nurse.

At school I have found the practical elements of Biology particularly fascinating and I enjoy learning how to use new equipment. I have specifically enjoyed learning about the functions of the human body and how different organs behave in health and disease. Keeping up to date with advances in medicine fascinates me and I regularly read the New Scientist. As a member of the school debating team I enjoy the opportunity to interact with a wide variety of people and discuss relevant current issues. Recently, for example, we had a lively debate about the recent MRSA problems and the reforms of the NHS to combat this. At the moment I am preparing a talk on 'Anorexia and the New Size 0' which I will be delivering to the debate team shortly; I am looking

forward to the opportunity to learn more about controversies such as this during my degree. By attending a Nurse Education Information session, I was able to listen to current Managers working in the NHS and increase my awareness of what training and a career in Nursing will involve, including the need for commitment to the continual updating of my skills and knowledge.

A part-time placement at a residential school for disabled children introduced me to the basics of providing personal care and the need for a sensitive and empathetic approach when dealing with patients and their families. This was useful experience for a subsequent short-term placement at a hospice in Ireland during which my duties were to chat to elderly patients. Here I learnt from the nurses about ethical issues such as patient confidentiality and autonomy. This placement was particularly intense as many of the patients were suffering from mental illnesses and could be very demanding. However, I felt inspired by the stamina and commitment shown by the staff and the experience reinforced my commitment to contributing to this field. Recently I gained a permanent position as a ward volunteer at a local hospital, which has been invaluable in giving me an understanding of how a hospital is run. My duties so far have involved befriending patients, helping to serve meals, assisting with personal care of patients and helping with clerical duties in the reception.

In my leisure time I enjoy sports and being captain of the local hockey team, which has won several tournaments, I have developed my strengths in leadership and teamwork through encouraging and supporting my team-mates. Through completing the Duke of Edinburgh silver award I have had the opportunity to learn a range of new skills, including playing the piano and organising fund raising events. As a senior prefect I enjoy contributing to my school community through supervising other prefects and providing pastoral care for younger members of the school. Taking a gap year will familiarise me with independent living and budgeting as I travel around South East Asia, preparing me for the transition from home to university. Before leaving I will be working in a supermarket for six months to save the money required, and I am confident that my gap year will be a useful chance to develop my maturity.

In conclusion, I am a self-motivated, enthusiastic and active student and I am confident that I have the skills and commitment required to achieve my goal of practising as an Adult Nurse within the NHS.

Character count: 3,712

Improving your Personal Statement

The following analysis aims to help you to create an engaging Personal Statement by looking at ways the 'draft' statement was refined. By considering the 'draft' and 'refined' paragraphs side by side, important principles can be highlighted.

Paragraph one: Draft

'I have always been interested in Adult Nursing so I would really like the chance to study this branch of Nursing at university. Two members of my family are both respected nurses and my ambition is to hold a similarly rewarding position in the community.'

Paragraph one: Refined

'Adult Nursing is a challenging and rewarding career that appeals to me as it combines my enjoyment of learning with my desire to contribute to improving people's health and wellbeing. As several of my relatives are nurses, I have benefited from discussions with them about the realities of a nursing career and about the need for communication skills and stamina in order to be a successful nurse.'

Paragraph one: Draft

The opening sentence is not particularly attention grabbing and does not give the admissions tutors any information beyond that the applicant wants to study Nursing; the admissions panel will have assumed this to be the case anyway.

39

Beware of claiming to have 'always' been interested in Nursing. Even if you did want to be a nurse at the age of three, you would not at that point have had the ability to make an informed decision on the subject. It can sound naïve to imply that you are applying to study a subject because it was your childhood dream, without demonstrating that you have since researched your future career fully. Ensure that you assign a capital letter to the name of the course i.e. Nursing not nursing.

In this paragraph there is no real justification for the applicant's interest in studying nursing. Remember that having a relative or family friend in nursing does not in itself improve the applicant's chances of gaining an interview. If the applicant feels that they have benefited from having frequent contact with a practising nurse, it is important that they show they have made use of this opportunity to learn more about the career.

In starting most sentences with 'I', the applicant shows a lack of written style, and this makes for a boring and uninspired Personal Statement, with the format lacking direction.

Paragraph one: Refined

By beginning the Personal Statement with a clear and well reasoned explanation of their reason for applying, the applicant makes a bold and engaging opening sentence and also shows that they have considered their career plans carefully. The influence of family members who are nurses is discussed and the applicant shows what they have learnt from this personal contact. This gives the impression that they are well informed about life as a nurse and that they are the type of person to make the most of opportunities around them.

Discussing qualities needed of a nurse suggests that the applicant has done their homework and investigated their career plans thoroughly. The more varied sentence structures keep the readers engaged and show that the applicant is capable of a more sophisticated writing style.

Paragraph two: Draft

'I have thoroughly enjoyed studying A level in Biology and I also enjoy reading other books about developments in Science and I believe I will enjoy studying Nursing at university. To explore the subject further I have been to the Nurse Education Information Afternoon at York University in 2009.'

Paragraph two: Refined

'At school I have found the practical elements of Biology particularly fascinating and I enjoy learning how to use new equipment. I have specifically enjoyed learning about the functions of the human body and how different organs behave in health and disease. Keeping up to date with advances in medicine fascinates me and I regularly read the New Scientist. As a member of the school debating team I enjoy the opportunity to interact with a wide variety of people and discuss relevant current issues. Recently, for example, we had a lively debate about the recent MRSA problems and the reforms of the NHS to combat this. At the moment I am preparing a talk on 'Anorexia and the New Size 0' which I will be delivering to the debate team shortly; I am looking forward to the opportunity to learn more about controversies such as this during my degree. By attending a Nurse Education Information session, I was able to listen to current Managers working in the NHS and increase my awareness of what training and a career in Nursing will involve, including the need for commitment to the continual updating of my skills and knowledge.'

Paragraph two: Draft

It is not necessary to repeat information, such as which A levels are being studied, which is given elsewhere on the UCAS form and doing so not only wastes valuable word space but also suggests the applicant has not thought out their Personal Statement thoroughly.

Although the applicant states that they enjoy Science, they have not given any examples to support this, and the tone of the paragraph is not particularly enthusiastic. This paragraph is your opportunity to show what you have learnt at school and what you have enjoyed about the learning process. The admissions tutors will be looking for people who are enthusiastic about the process of studying Nursing at their university for several years, as well as being enthusiastic about practising as a nurse later.

Although it is mentioned that the applicant likes books about Science this is not supported by any examples and there is no indication of what they have learnt from this. The applicant then states that they have attended a Nurse Education Information session, but again does not explain what they have learnt or gained from the experience. Again, remember that many of your fellow applicants will have attended similar sessions; it is up to you to show how this experience has made you a better candidate.

It is also important not to waste your word limit giving too much irrelevant detail. For example, the admissions tutors do not need to know the location of the seminars you have attended. This paragraph adds very little to the Personal Statement and the applicant misses an opportunity to show how they have prepared themselves for the academic rigour of a Nursing degree.

Paragraph two: Refined

The applicant goes into much greater detail about what they have learnt from their academic experience over the last couple of years. By discussing the elements of their subject which they have enjoyed they are highlighting their skills in and enthusiasm for Science as well as demonstrating an awareness of how A level Biology has helped them to prepare for degree level study.

By mentioning relevant journals and current issues in nursing which they are aware of, the applicant shows not only that they are reading outside their schoolwork but also what they are learning from this. Discussing what they have gained from the Nurse Education Information session has the same effect.

The section regarding the debate team has been moved to this paragraph as it is most relevant here. As well as knowledge of topics related to nursing, this is an opportunity to demonstrate that you have learnt wider academic skills such as conducting self-directed research and delivering presentations.

Paragraph three: Draft

'I have also taken on some work experience in a range of nursing areas. I started in 2005 working at Hope House near Reading, which is a residential school for disabled children. I worked there every Wednesday and Saturday afternoon for two years during term-time. Last summer, I went with a group to Ireland for a week to work in a hospice as a volunteer looking after some of the patients there. This was a very demanding experience but it did not discourage me, rather it was one of the most amazing experiences of my life and I plan to return next year. I have also recently started a permanent position as a ward volunteer at Reading District General Hospital. I have also discussed my future career with family members who work in nursing, and I am confident that I am well suited to this career.'

Paragraph three: Refined

'A part-time placement at a residential school for disabled children introduced me to the basics of providing personal care and the need for a sensitive and empathetic approach when dealing with patients and their families. This was useful experience for a subsequent short-term placement at a hospice in Ireland during which my duties were to chat to elderly patients. Here I learnt from the nurses about ethical issues such as patient confidentiality and autonomy. This placement was particularly intense as many of the patients were suffering from mental illnesses and could be very demanding. However, I felt inspired by the stamina and

---

> *commitment shown by the staff and the experience reinforced my commitment to contributing to this field. Recently I gained a permanent position as a ward volunteer at a local hospital, which has been invaluable in giving me an understanding of how a hospital is run. My duties so far have involved befriending patients, helping to serve meals, assisting with personal care of patients and helping with clerical duties in the reception.'*

Paragraph three: Draft

This paragraph reads too much as if the applicant has simply listed all the relevant experience that they have had. With no reflection on what they have gained from this, they are not making the most of the opportunity to discuss how these experiences have influenced their decision to study Nursing. Relevant work experience is one of the key areas in which you can make your application stand out from the competition.

There is also too much space wasted with irrelevant details such as precise names and locations and the days in which the applicant worked there, which add nothing to the strength of the application. In referring to the placement in Ireland the applicant has said that it was *'one of the most amazing experiences of my life'*, a strong statement but with no indication of why the experience was so 'amazing', or why it is relevant to their application. The paragraph ends with an unrelated sentence that should have been included in the first paragraph, with the other mention of the family members.

Paragraph three: Refined

This paragraph now forms a key part of the Personal Statement, showing the breadth of experience the applicant has and how it has helped them to decide on a career in nursing. There are no unnecessary details and the applicant explains precisely what their duties were and what they have gained from this, both in terms of practical skills such as personal care and wider issues such as confidentiality. The placement in Ireland is discussed in more detail and it is now clear why the applicant found it challenging but also inspiring.

Paragraph four: Draft

'I am a keen member of the school debating team and I am also captain of the hockey team, which has won several local tournaments. My involvement in the debating team has given me the chance to meet new people and develop skills in team working. Whilst playing in the hockey team has given me the chance to develop leadership skills and keep fit. I have also been involved in other extra-curricular activities through completing the Duke of Edinbourgh silver award. I am also a senior prefect. Art is another hobby of mine, and I like to visit various art galleries in my holidays. I love travelling and I have been to Canada, the USA, France, Italy and Spain. For this reason, I jumped at the chance of a gap year, and I will be working in Britain for six months before I set off travelling.'

Paragraph four: Refined

'In my leisure time I enjoy sports and being captain of the local hockey team, which has won several tournaments, I have developed my strengths in leadership and teamwork through encouraging and supporting my team-mates. Through completing the Duke of Edinburgh silver award I have had the opportunity to learn a range of new skills, including playing the piano and organising fund raising events. As a senior prefect I enjoy contributing to my school community through supervising other prefects and providing pastoral care for younger members of the school. Taking a gap year will familiarise me with independent living and budgeting as I travel around South East Asia, preparing me for the transition from home to university. Before leaving I will be working in a supermarket for six months to save the money required, and I am confident that my gap year will be a useful chance to develop my maturity.'

Paragraph four: Draft

The incorrect spelling of Edinburgh shows, at best, someone who does not take care in their writing and, at worst, someone who has poor spelling! Make sure that all spelling and grammar is correct; small mistakes will make a big (and bad) impression.

The language is unadventurous, and the applicant rushes through things in a list-like fashion, which minimises the importance and impact of their achievements. It is far better to mention one or two hobbies or achievements and demonstrate how these have helped you to develop useful skills than to attempt to list everything that interests you. Think carefully about which of your hobbies are relevant. Being captain of a sports team is clearly a great opportunity to show that you are familiar with working within a team of people, a vital skill for a career in nursing. The short, rushed sentence about art can be taken out completely as it is not relevant to the application and wastes valuable space.

Listing destinations visited risks sounding as though you are showing off and unless you have taken part in some daring expedition or learnt a new language whilst abroad, listing your family's holiday destinations will not impress the admissions panel. Taking a gap year can be an asset to an application, but only if you can show that you have given it thought and do not just want to take a break for a year.

Paragraph four: Refined

Here the applicant lists only those hobbies that can be justified as relevant to their application. Details are given as to how being the captain of the hockey team and involvement in the Duke of Edinburgh award have helped them to develop and mature, showing the applicant to be a well-rounded person.

The requirements of being a senior prefect are given and the paragraph points to the contributions the student may make to the university community. In their discussion of their gap year the applicant shows that they have planned a structured year and suggests they have chosen to take a year out for their personal growth, as preparation for university rather than as a way of avoiding it.

Concluding paragraph: Draft

Does not exist.

Concluding paragraph: Refined

'In conclusion, I am a self-motivated, enthusiastic and active student and I am confident that I have the skills and commitment required to achieve my goal of practising as an Adult Nurse within the NHS.'

Concluding paragraph: Draft

A concluding paragraph is absolutely imperative in order to leave the reader with your most important reasons for gaining a place on your chosen course. It is a huge mistake not to include one, as it will mean that your Personal Statement will tail off, leaving the reader feeling that you have no real focus.

Concluding paragraph: Refined

The start of the paragraph gives a hint that the Personal Statement is nearly finished, giving the reader time to reconsider the points the applicant has made – it may also provide relief for weary admissions tutors! The applicant gives a broad summary of their academic *and* social skills, emphasising both their academic interest but also their well-rounded personality (this is not the time to introduce new information).

Key points

The 'draft' and 'refined' versions of this fictitious example are presented in order to illustrate the principles underpinning the preparation of a compelling Personal Statement.

Your Personal Statement must describe **you**; **your** personal qualities, **your** enthusiasms, **your** strengths.

Make sure the material you present in your Personal Statement really does convince the reader that you have a very good idea of what you are getting into, that studying Nursing is right for you, **and** that you are right for the nursing profession.

Chapter 7

Personal Statement examples for applying to Nursing

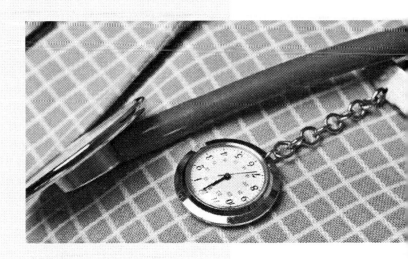

Personal Statement examples for applying to Nursing

Example 1

Nursing appeals to me as a demanding but rewarding profession which integrates theory and practice in promoting the health and well-being of patients. After a change of career direction I have worked as a hospital Nursing Auxiliary for two years and now wish to take the next step in my progress towards becoming a Registered Nurse. As well as practising my profession I am interested in the structure and running of the NHS and hope to make a significant contribution to the development of this institution.

Studying on an Access to Health Studies course has been a thoroughly enjoyable return to education, particularly the chance to discuss projects with tutors and other students. Human Biology has given me a basic understanding of body systems, and cell and tissue structure, including practical experience of dissecting a sheep's internal organs which I found very interesting. Perspectives on Health Care has been the most exciting module, examining the social and psychological factors influencing a person's health from infancy to old age. During my Nursing degree I look forward to enhancing these studies as well as my practical skills during clinical placements. In particular, I am interested in studying Social Theory and Public Health, exploring the social implications of inequalities of health and the role of preventative methods in health promotion.

Working as a Nursing Auxiliary in an acute paediatric ward has allowed me to learn a great deal about a nurse's daily duties and workload. Having witnessed many traumatic situations, including the delivery of tragic news to families, I feel I will be embarking on a career in Nursing with a realistic appreciation of both the challenges and rewards of the profession. My duties include personal care, grooming, feeding and comforting patients as well as organising medicines and maintaining detailed patient records. I have also been involved in a committee charged with supervising the implementation of the new Working Time Directive. As a Health and Safety Officer, I have a further level of responsibility and I have enjoyed these opportunities to play an active part in the hospital community. My job has developed in me strong interpersonal skills and the ability to work well in a multi-disciplinary team delivering the best possible patient care. I have an appreciation of the role of different health and social care professionals and I wish to specialise as a Child Health Nurse.

Outside work, I enjoy my involvement with Guides, as a pack leader helping to encourage and support young women as they grow up. This involves weekly meetings and two trips abroad each year. As well as leadership skills and experience with children and parents, I have developed proficiency in administration and time management, and strong critical skills when assessing the Health and Safety risks and requirements of our trips abroad. In leisure time, I enjoy rock climbing and am a qualified Mountain Leader, which required two years of preparation, training and assessment. This sport has taken me around the world, including a recent expedition to the Peruvian Andes. As well as the chance to test and develop my abilities, I make the most of these opportunities to discover new cultures, languages and landscapes.

My employment experience has confirmed that I am suited to a career in nursing and I am fully committed to enhancing my prospects for career development. After registering as a Child Health Nurse, I hope to continue to train to the highest level and look forward to playing a full role as an NHS practitioner.

Example 2

Since completing my work experience in a hospice for people with terminal illness, I have been committed to pursuing a career in nursing. My A level Biology has provided me with a background in the science of the human body and I have enjoyed learning about the functions and interactions of the different systems. My coursework investigating the functions of proteins on plants and animals has been very interesting and has allowed me to develop my research skills. In Chemistry I have again found the practical work very engaging, especially the challenge of collating everyone's results to draw a conclusion during group research.

Three weeks of work experience at a hospice was very influential in my decision to apply for Nursing and taught me the daily reality of caring for people who may be distressed, uncomfortable and frightened. During my time there one of the elderly residents died, which was upsetting for me but I felt inspired by the professional yet compassionate manner with which the staff dealt with the lady in question and with her grieving family. To confirm my suitability for nursing I have since obtained a part-time job as a Ward Assistant in a busy general hospital. This has given me the opportunity to work within the ward team ensuring our section is run smoothly and our patients can receive the best possible care. This job has taught me a great deal about the importance of hygiene as well as the roles of the different professionals and how they interact. During night shifts I am the supervisor, with responsibility for ensuring all the ward assistants' duties are completed according to the schedule and writing a concise shift report for the handover at the end of the shift. These extra duties have allowed me to develop my interpersonal and leadership skills and increased my confidence when dealing with colleagues and the public.

Working in a hospital and observing treatments being administered around me has captured my curiosity and I am very excited about learning all aspects of Nursing during my degree. In particular, I have an interest in public health, which has received a great deal of press recently due to the problems with MRSA, and how to best manage care and treatment within complex multiple environments. Related topics such as healthcare law and ethics also interest me and I enjoy following such issues in the broadsheet newspapers. The clinical placements, with the opportunity to implement and enhance my interpersonal skills, will be excellent practise for the working environment and I also look forward to the opportunity to debate subjects with other students across the healthcare programmes.

As a Senior Prefect at school I have been responsible for organising a team of eight Prefects and assisting the staff in the smooth running of the school. This has further developed my leadership qualities and I enjoy making a responsible contribution to the school. For the last five years I have competed at national level in water skiing, representing my region first in the Junior section and now in the Adult competitions. Competing at this level requires frequent training and a great deal of self-discipline in order to improve my ability. This year I have been selected for the national team and will be competing at the World Championships in Tokyo, where I hope to be placed at least third. I also enjoy other water sports such as wind surfing and sailing and I intend to be involved in adventure sports societies at university. I am a highly motivated student with interests in many areas and a genuine commitment to a career as a nurse and I look forward to making the most of the opportunities available to me at university.

Example 3

Since training as a cosmetician I have had the ambition of one day pursuing a career in healthcare. Nursing particularly appeals to me as it offers huge variety and scope for interaction with people from all walks of life, with great opportunities for future career development and specialisation. A career in this field would be challenging and rewarding, and my determination to make a positive contribution to the Health Service has led me to apply to study Adult Nursing.

In Germany I worked in a Dermatology surgery as a cosmetician for two and a half years. This involved manning the reception, taking phone calls, dealing with patients' enquiries and typing medical reports. It also gave me my first taste of patient care through assisting the doctor in operations, botox and laser treatments. After appropriate training I performed laser hair-removal, wart treatments, allergy tests and the preparation of immunisation injections independently. Much of the job involved advising and supporting patients, for example, helping teenage acne sufferers feel better about their appearance and informing them about cover-up make up and other options. I also acted as deputy manager in the absence of my boss on several occasions, giving me experience of running the business and taking overall responsibility for patient care and for the presentation and hygiene of the surgery. Since returning to work after having my daughter I have been working for a contract cleaning company at the Walsall Primary Care Trust. Although this does not involve direct patient care I have enjoyed contact with patients and have taken the opportunity to learn more about the daily workings of an NHS hospital and the roles of different health professionals. My employment experience has given me knowledge of the role of a nurse and the qualities required of healthcare workers as well as excellent interpersonal skills, with the ability to inform, instruct and advise people on all levels.

Personal experiences have also motivated me to change careers. At the age of 28, my partner had a near-fatal motorcycle accident and I became his full-time carer until he returned to work two years later. This experience changed my perception of life as I learnt to distinguish between trivialities and genuinely important things and to put the needs of others before my own. As well as a range of practical skills associated with caring, I gained an insight into the effect of illness on carers and loved ones and the need for empathy and support as a nurse when dealing with patients' families. The support of the nurses when my daughter was born two months prematurely was further demonstration of the importance of their role and confirmed my desire to study this subject. During my cosmetician training the areas of anatomy, physiology and dermatology particularly fascinated me, and I am especially looking forward to studying the theoretical aspects of these subjects during my degree, as well as gaining practical experience of different procedures.

As a teenager, I competed at national level in trampolining, receiving many medals and awards. This sport is still a passion of mine, and I am now involved in coaching beginners and as a qualified competition judge. I am also currently studying for the European Computer Driving Licence, which will consolidate my IT knowledge. After qualifying as a nurse I hope to continue my training throughout my career, and to specialise either in the environment of an operating theatre or a dermatology ward. I am fully committed to practising as a nurse and I feel I have the skills and motivation necessary to succeed both during my training and in my future career.

Example 4

My motivation to train as a nurse stems from my desire to utilise my academic and interpersonal skills in a role which will allow me to contribute positively to people's quality of life. Extensive work experience with people with social problems has confirmed my interest in opting for the Learning Disability branch in the second year and I look forward to gaining the knowledge and practical training required to begin nursing in this field.

At school I have particularly enjoyed Biology A level, which has given me a useful background in human physiology and anatomy. The range of skills utilised in this subject, such as qualitative and quantitative research, report writing, technical drawing and making poster presentations has been very engaging and I look forward to the variety of learning methods offered by a degree in Nursing. Chemistry has further developed my ability in both group and independent research and I found our experiments creating aspirins and learning about the effects of drugs on the body very interesting. In Media Studies I have developed my powers of critical analysis and evaluation as well as my written, verbal and creative communication skills. I believe these will be valuable assets when required to inform patients, families and staff, who will all have different levels of understanding, about treatment procedures.

My first work experience placement was at a residential special needs school for primary age children with learning and behavioural difficulties. This was an enlightening experience and I felt inspired by the work of the teachers, nurses and support staff who put so much effort into encouraging and motivating the pupils. After this placement I secured a part-time job at the school as a support assistant which involves helping the staff in delivering outdoor activities for the pupils. This has the challenge of the extra safety requirements of the less mobile pupils and their widely differing educational needs. Two further work placements, shadowing a psychiatric nurse in a hospital and the receptionist of a busy A&E ward, have given me experience of the hospital environment and allowed me to learn about the NHS. I have enjoyed the opportunity to discuss topical issues with the hospital staff, such as the current debate regarding patient choice in the allocation of single rooms.

As a Beat Bullying Mentor at school, I attend weekly meetings and help to organise workshops between bullies and victims as part of an initiative to combat this problem by involving the pupils in the process. I have also worked as a camp counsellor on a PGL activity holiday for children with learning difficulties, which has developed my confidence in dealing with people with disabilities and reinforced my belief that it is important to remain open-minded as to an individual's capabilities and potential. Having played the violin for several years, I have learned the importance of persistence and focus when practising for performances and am currently preparing for my Grade 7 exam. I also enjoy singing with the choir and participating in the Debating Society, both of which I would like to continue at university. After graduation, I hope to become a Registered Nurse and then to specialise as a nurse in learning disabilities. I believe that a career in this field will be extremely rewarding and I look forward to the challenges and opportunities of university.

Example 5

The opportunity to be able to make a difference to people's lives has always been at the forefront of my career aspirations. Indeed, I have been interested in the healthcare profession since I was a child, but due to financial hardship within my family and the social problems that this has caused, I failed to achieve the necessary qualifications at school. The birth of my last child has precipitated my return to education in order to realise my ambition and dream; it has been caring for him that reminded me of my childhood aspirations. The support of the midwives and nurses has made me more determined to achieve my goal.

In 2007, I decided to match my interest and ambition to my skills and enrol for the Pre-Access to Science Study. I am currently completing an Access to Nursing and Midwifery course to develop and improve my knowledge and skills in a range of subjects including Biology, Chemistry, Mathematics, English, IT and Study Skills. I believe this shows my determination to gain admission to university, despite not having achieved the conventional qualifications necessary. I also feel that this course has helped me to develop my ability to communicate effectively with a variety of people, to successfully meet deadlines and to cope in stressful situations, all skills I believe will benefit me in my future carer as a nurse.

As a mother of three, I enjoy working with my children and supporting them with their school assignments. I make particular effort to work closely with their schools to improve their performance and progress. In addition, I work voluntarily as a co-ordinator for the youth section of my church. My role involves organising, planning and coordinating programmes, collaborating with other youth clubs in the community, taking part in exhibitions, competitions, festivals and song revivals. I also fundraise for the local care home and Children in Need. These roles have improved my ability to take a thoughtful and logical approach to problem solving.

Working as a care assistant, I have enhanced my knowledge of the needs of patients and their relatives in a particularly stressful situation. My duties include personal care of the patient, bathing, feeding and laundry. While at work, I am responsible for informing and reporting any changes in the condition of the patient to the Social Care Liaison Team as well as maintaining confidentiality and attending training sessions to upgrade my knowledge, so as to meet the standards and expectations of patient care. These duties have given me more experience, helped me to cope with difficult situations by using my initiative and helped me to be more sympathetic and more concerned about the well being and feelings of others. In spite of my duties, I am able to keep my work and family commitment in balance.

In my spare time, I enjoy reading about current affairs, and folktales with my children, and cooking multicultural dishes. I am confident that I will be a dedicated and diligent student, and studying at your institution will equip and prepare me for a successful career in nursing.

Example 6

My ambition has always been to pursue a career in which I can work closely with people in a nurturing environment and where I can make a positive impact on their lives. Following school, my training in the beauty profession gave me the opportunity to work with people, interacting on a personal level and responding to their needs, but I felt I needed to expand my horizons and face new challenges. A career in nursing had always been a dream of mine, so with this in mind I made the decision to move from hairdressing to take up a job as a Care Assistant at a residential home for the elderly in order to appreciate, first hand, the demands of working in a healthcare environment. From this experience I realised that I not only loved taking care of vulnerable people and learning to become sensitive to their individual needs, but that I thrived in this busy and demanding environment and enjoyed being a valuable member of the healthcare team.

With renewed determination to follow a career as a nurse I successfully applied to the NHS for a job as a Nursing Assistant, which I held for two years, before taking up my current position as a Clinical Support Nurse. During this time I have gained a wealth of practical expertise related to nursing care as well as developing the personal skills I believe are essential to nursing, namely excellent communication and teamwork skills combined with the ability to provide care for patients in a way which shows respect and empathy while preserving their dignity and individuality. Although this work is physically and mentally challenging I find it immensely rewarding and it has given me a valuable insight into the demands that are required from a healthcare professional.

In the last five years I have also learned how to organise my time effectively so that I am able to combine working the required shift patterns with taking time to study for essential qualifications that I believe will benefit my career. As well as gaining an NVQ in perioperative care, I decided to commit further to my career by funding myself in order to study for recognised OCN and OCR qualifications, and complete two Open University modules in health- and medical-related topics, successfully gaining 75 OU credits. As an added benefit I learnt to use up-to-date word-processing facilities and information technology in order to research and present my written assignments, and this helped me to develop the computer and IT skills that I now apply to my job on a daily basis. Studying for these qualifications has given me confidence in my ability to complete tasks under demanding circumstances and shows I am hard working, conscientious and committed to my goal.

I strongly believe it is important to find a balance between the demands of work and recreational and social interests. I therefore enjoy being involved in family activities and, as a mother, encourage outdoor and social pursuits as well as keeping myself physically fit through horse riding, cycling and gymnastics. I am excited about the prospect of studying for a Nursing Diploma at Exeter University and believe I am well prepared for the challenges I will face. I consider myself to be a reliable, dedicated and responsible person with a mature approach and a passion to succeed in my chosen vocation as a career nurse.

Example 7

My desire for a stimulating career through which I can help to make a positive difference to people's quality of life has motivated me to apply for Nursing. This has been reinforced by extensive work experience in a range of healthcare environments which has confirmed my dedication to pursuing this career. Through my school work I have developed a proven ability to manage my time and resources efficiently to meet tight deadlines, and to maintain a consistently high standard. Knowing that nursing is highly demanding I have researched it thoroughly and, as a naturally positive person with a sense of humour and a wide range of non-academic pursuits, I feel I have the coping strategies necessary to deal with the pressures of a Nursing degree and career.

As part of the Monklands Next Generation Programme, I have visited departments including A&E, Cardiology and a Diabetes Clinic, learning about the structure of the hospital and the complementary roles played by different members of the team. Attending sessions of Breastfeeding and Child Immunisation Clinics highlighted the importance of prevention as part of successful healthcare provision, and also added to my awareness of the difficult and controversial issues within nursing. I have spent time shadowing a Cardiologist Nurse and a Community Nurse attending Child Development Clinics. This has allowed me to see many of the different career paths available and their demanding daily routines. I made use of the opportunity to learn as much as possible about a career in nursing and observed the need for empathy, stamina and dedication across all areas. Having also spent time in a Libyan hospital, at a Burns Clinic for outpatients, I have been able to compare the different health systems and appreciate what the NHS can offer.

At school I was a senior member of the Health Awareness Committee, organising and delivering campaigns in healthy eating and smoking awareness. This involved liaising with members of the team, and motivating and supporting others. At the Autism Unit I helped support children with autism and Asperger's Syndrome to achieve their best, and I also acted as a mentor in the 'buddy system', and worked as a classroom assistant with first year pupils. Regular babysitting jobs have shown me the importance of being patient and creative when dealing with children; my first aid skills also prove useful when dealing with minor injuries. During my gap year I am a volunteer at a nursing home where I am learning about the particular needs of the elderly and experiencing hands-on primary care. I am also continuing my work as a Samaritan. Here I take calls from severely troubled people and have received training in the listening skills and non-judgemental manner which is required to help the callers. This work appeals to my empathetic nature and has given me an insight into mental health problems. In these environments, as well as helping in a charity shop, I am developing excellent communication and interpersonal skills with a diversity of patients, families, customers and colleagues.

At school I was on the newspaper team, writing articles and helping to sell issues. This provided a great creative outlet and I continue to write short stories and poetry. When the Scottish weather permits, I enjoy hill-walking and landscape photography. Developing my images using Photoshop software I also create avatars, wallpapers, and music videos. I play in a local netball club and go jogging most weekends, and am currently teaching myself Arabic dancing. In an effort to expand my communicative potential and to prepare myself for my continental travels, I am also learning French.

I am fully committed to my aim of becoming a successful nurse, providing the best possible care for my patients and I believe I have the skills and motivation to achieve my goals.

Example 8

Having found my current career unfulfilling for several years it has been a longstanding ambition to pursue a career in the provision of primary health care. Nursing appeals to me as it offers a great deal of variety and scope for interaction with patients from all backgrounds and health and social care professionals from many disciplines. A career in this field would be extremely rewarding and give me the opportunity to develop my skills in a specialised area.

For the last ten years I have worked in administration, having been unable to enter university straight after school due to financial constraints. Although I have progressed well within my company, I have found it insufficiently stimulating and with little scope for promotion or professional development. Now that my children are at school and I have the full support of my family, I am confident that the time is right to commit to returning to education and pursuing a career in nursing.

For the last four years I have been employed as a personal carer for a severely disabled young woman which has taught me a great deal about the skills required of a good nurse. My duties include all aspects of personal care and grooming, feeding, preparing medication and transporting my client to appointments. Once a week, I also cover the night shift, and I maintain detailed records of each shift to pass on to the next carer. As well as the practical skills involved, this has taught me how to manage my time efficiently, remain constantly alert and maintain a professional and compassionate manner in all circumstances. I have also been able to observe the role of the team of medical professionals assigned to her care, and the experiences of her family, which are an important element of her well being. Undertaking a three-week work placement shadowing a Community

Nurse on her rounds has been very useful; demonstrating the variety of her cases and familiarising me with a typical daily routine. Next month I will be spending two weeks shadowing a nurse based in the A&E Department which will provide an interesting contrast and allow me to learn more about the NHS system.

My employment with my present company has involved a range of secretarial and administrative jobs which have provided me with many transferable skills. My current role is as Retail Project Support, working as part of a team providing customer service to all internal staff, clients and customers. Supporting the Project Managers requires me to be well organised, confident and have the ability to communicate well with everyone and to prioritise my workload. Taking minutes of meetings, organising daily correspondence, and producing monthly reports has given me highly effective written and verbal communication skills. My employment has enabled me to interact with people on all levels and has given me the ability to work in a team. I also have the confidence to take initiative in difficult situations and to have an open-minded approach to problem solving.

In leisure time I enjoy keeping active by swimming with my children and have recently joined a local singing group which I thoroughly enjoy and find to have a very calming and positive effect. As a mature applicant I have carefully researched my possible career paths and as a practical individual with a caring nature I feel I have the qualities required to fulfil my ambition of becoming an efficient and compassionate nursing professional.

Example 9

My desire to study Nursing stems from my experience in my current career as a carer. While I enjoy the role of helping people, I find myself feeling constricted by the limitations placed on me in the job. Recently, I have become increasingly frustrated that I am not able to do more for patients when I have identified any additional needs they may have. It is for this reason that I would like to change my focus to nursing, and ultimately realise my ambition of specialising in Community Nursing. I look forward to studying all aspects of the subject at university, but I am especially keen to learn more about the application of knowledge and skills in acute adult care.

I firmly believe that my career as a carer will hold me in good stead for my time studying and practising nursing, and give me an advantage as I already have a fair amount of medical knowledge and experience to draw upon. Having worked closely with elderly, disabled and memory impaired patients, I have developed the skills of empathy and compassion to a high degree, as well as being able to understand the needs of those who might not be able to communicate them effectively themselves. The role also involves liaising with patients' families, social services and other health organisations, as well as co-workers, so effective communication skills are essential. As I work closely with nurses on a daily basis, I have developed the essential skill of being able to work as part of a team, while retaining the ability to think and make decisions independently. Having also discussed this career choice with my mother, a District Nursing Manager, she gave me the opportunity to shadow her at work for a day, affording me a greater insight into what the details and duties of her position entail. Having sought her advice and gained her approval, coupled with my experience of working in the community, I am absolutely certain that nursing is my ideal career.

As I have experience myself of suffering from a long-term illness in ME, I believe I am better equipped than most to understand what patients are going through. Additionally, my grandmother passed away very recently in a sudden accident, which really gave me the impetus to pursue my goal of studying Nursing, because it made me realise the need to make the most of any opportunities we get in our short lifetimes.

I understand the importance of good time-management when it comes to studying and the necessity of having a good work/pleasure balance. To this end I enjoy creative and calming activities like meditation and photography; I would like to carry on with these at university as they will be a great outlet for the stresses and pressures of studying for a Diploma. To relax I intend to pursue my other passions, including attending the theatre, reading, painting and socialising with friends and family. I am confident that these extra-curricular activities will help me to succeed at university, as well as contributing to life on campus.

In summation, I would like to emphasise my passion for the field and the way that my previous experiences as a carer will aid me well in my studies. I will make a dedicated, conscientious and committed student who has a good support base in family and friends, and extra-curricular activities which will help to alleviate any stress. Studying for a Diploma in Nursing will give me the opportunity to realise my ambitions and it is for this reason that I am certain I will succeed at university.

Example 10

The options available to a nurse interest me greatly, and the different spheres within which they operate, such as the hospital and community, provide the job variation which I crave. It has long since been my ambition to be a part of the lives of others, where I can offer my support and advice; I feel a career as a nurse would provide me this opportunity.

Biology has been one of my favourite subjects within my Access Course as I enjoy learning about human anatomy and physiology. I have also made the most of this opportunity to practise my study skills to ensure I am able to make the most of my degree. At university I am looking forward to learning general aspects of nursing prior to specialisation in Children's Nursing. Within this subject, I am particularly looking forward to developing my ability to interpret the behaviour of children in order to assess the nature and severity of their suffering, helping to ease it accordingly. My Access Course has included two weeks of work experience in a hospital which was an excellent chance to connect theory with practice and I am very excited about undertaking clinical placements when learning how to care for both children and their families. At college I have enjoyed investigating research projects and learning to assimilate large quantities of information. I am excited about taking my return to education to a higher level and look forward to the challenge of continuing to update my knowledge throughout my career.

My employment history has given me many transferable skills which will be useful during my training and future career. As a call centre supervisor for a large Internet Service Provider I manage a team of seven and deal with the more difficult queries or complaints as they are referred to me. This requires effective interpersonal skills in order to get the necessary information from the caller, and to determine and solve their problem. Calls come from people of all ages and levels of ability in English and in IT and I feel my experience of this, as well as my fluency in three languages, will be valuable in multi-ethnic communities. My job frequently involves dealing with angry and unpleasant customers with a calm and professional approach and I am familiar with working in a pressurised environment. Using different software packages to give advice to callers on the helpline, computers are an integral part of my working day and I have also been able to develop good organisational and time management skills.

Volunteering with the St. John Ambulance service, including Advanced First Aid training, has confirmed my enjoyment of working in healthcare. It has also given me some basic medical knowledge and inspired me to learn more. In order to further my experience I will soon be starting a part-time job as a First Aider within St. John Ambulance Caring Services. Training with St. John Ambulance has taught me the value of commitment and dedication, as well as providing experience of working as a team to reach common goals. Prior to my most recent job I was employed in customer services by Marks and Spencer. A substantial part of this job was training staff, many of them significantly older than me, on the new computer systems.

My work with the St. John Ambulance Service has confirmed that I am suited to a job in the caring professions. As a mature applicant I have had the time to fully research and consider my options and I feel I am particularly suited to nursing. My ambition is to work as a qualified nurse within the NHS, making a significant contribution to the provision of high quality patient care, and I feel I have the commitment and motivation required to achieve my goal.

Example 11

Since completing a work experience placement shadowing a community-based nurse for three weeks, and finding the role to be varied, stimulating and rewarding, I have had an ambition to study Nursing at university.

At school I have found Biology A level a particularly interesting subject as I am fascinated by the anatomy and physiology of the human body. Practical classes have always been my favourite as I enjoy learning from hands-on experience. As such I have found experiments in Biology and Chemistry, such as making aspirin and studying the growth of different bacteria, very exciting. English A level has been an opportunity to develop a different approach to study, and I have especially enjoyed the insight into other cultures which our range of literature has given me. Having studied both science and arts subjects at A level I have strong communication skills and a logical approach to problem solving. I have enjoyed opportunities to work in pairs and groups as I find it beneficial to discuss issues with others.

During my time at university I am looking forward to the range of disciplines which are covered in Nursing, and to the blocks of practical experience which will allow me to practise clinical skills before starting my career. My work experience placement introduced me to many aspects of the nurse's role and I look forward to putting this in an academic context. In particular, the importance of effective communication skills with both patients and the many other healthcare professionals the nurse interacted with was demonstrated. For the last year I have worked at the weekends and during school holidays as a care assistant at a nursing home, talking to patients and helping the nurses to care for them and administer their medicines. This has given me an appreciation of some of the different careers available in healthcare, as well as experience of interacting in an empathetic and sensitive manner with patients and of working within a team of assistants.

From the age of five I have spent much of my leisure time training and performing in ballet and modern dance, and have competed many times at national level, most recently winning the silver medal at the British Under-18s Dance finals. As a dancer I am responsible for managing myself as a performer, ensuring I maintain my fitness levels, devising my timetable and meeting potential agents and employees. This has given me skills in self-motivation, discipline and time management. Dancing remains an important part of my life and I hope to continue performing at university, setting up or running dance clubs and organising performances. I have performed in the West End, toured Austria and Italy, and have also coached children up to the age of twelve voluntarily at a ballet school. I am a motivated and disciplined student, with a range of active interests and a strong commitment to working as a nurse. This degree will equip me well for my future career and I feel I have the qualities to be able to make the most of the opportunities available to me at university

Example 12

In training to be a nurse, I hope to put my compassionate manner and enjoyment of working with others to good use by helping to alleviate patients' suffering. Having worked as a Ward Clerk for several years, I have an appreciation of what the job entails and the requirements of a good nurse. For the past two years I have studied a part-time Access Course to prepare myself academically for my degree and I now wish to take the next step on my new career path by taking a Nursing degree.

Working as a Ward Clerk has been a useful introduction to the hospital environment. In my day to day work I deal with patients, visitors, health and social care workers, executives and support staff with a friendly and professional manner, and have learned about the different roles of these people. As I am based in Neonatal Intensive Care, my job includes updating the patient information records each morning, organising medication requests from the pharmacy, assisting parents who are staying on-site, answering phone calls, booking appointments and organising the repair and maintenance of the ward facilities. This work has given me inside knowledge of how an NHS Trust is run and has shown me the difficult aspects of nursing such as dealing with the deaths of babies and grieving families. Using the hospital computer system as an integral part of my job has developed in me confident ICT skills which I will be able to make use of both during my degree and in my future work. As a Ward Clerk I do my best to make people's experience of hospital less stressful but I look forward to being able to make a real difference to patients' quality of treatment as a nurse.

During my Access Course I have especially enjoyed the modules on Science and Prevention of Infection as these have allowed me to make use of my employment background to add context to the theory. Communications has also been an interesting part of the course and I feel skill in this area is one of the most important qualities in a good nurse. At university I hope to build on my academic knowledge and learn how to put research into practice during clinical placements. At this stage I am planning to follow the Mental Health route and I am particularly interested in studying the sociological and psychological aspects of effective patient care.

In leisure time I enjoy my position on a local football team which is currently top of our league. Regular team training provides excellent exercise and I enjoy meeting players from all walks of life. As the club's social secretary I put my organisational skills to good use arranging fundraising and team building events such as karaoke nights and pub quizzes. I also enjoy staying up to date with current issues in nursing by reading journals such as the Nursing Times. Applying to study Nursing is a personal challenge for me and I hope to make the most of this opportunity to prove my academic ability and to improve my career prospects. I am embarking on a nursing career with a realistic awareness of what it entails and I look forward to taking on its rewards and challenges.

Example 13

Ever since I was nine years old and met my friend David, who had Down's syndrome, I have been inspired to work with, and help, people with special needs. Although I had always dreamed of becoming a nurse, being a young, single mother to my daughter, I decided to concentrate on supporting us both; holding down a full-time job until I was financially secure enough to pursue my Nursing studies. Now, with my marriage planned for February, and with the help and support of my fiancé and family, I feel that it is the perfect time to focus on my future career as a nurse and so apply to study on the three-year Nursing degree.

As a first step towards this goal I am currently studying full-time on the 'Access to Nursing' course at Bridgend College, while also working for my National Vocational Qualification level 3 in Health Care. I am finding this course extremely interesting, as not only does it build upon what I learnt through my National Vocational Qualification level 2 in Business Studies and my GCSE English, it is also enormously helpful and relevant to my current job in Brynawel House, an alcohol rehabilitation centre. Having gained valuable work placement experience in the past with mentally ill patients I enjoy my current responsibilities, working within this community to look after adults with combined learning disabilities and problems with alcohol abuse. Although the job is challenging and sometimes stressful I find the work very rewarding, particularly when making sure clients refrain from alcohol, assessing their needs, drawing up care plans and detailing their needs and abilities, including risk assessments, to ensure they receive the best possible care. As an organised person I enjoy being in charge of planning activities and holidays, working as part of a team with qualified staff and social welfare professionals to make sure that my clients live their lives as fully as possible, whilst respecting their dignity and rights.

Over the last ten years I have developed a wide range of clinical, interpersonal and communication skills through a broad and varied range of work placements. Having a positive attitude to working with people with behavioural problems, I greatly enjoyed the challenge of working with both elderly mentally ill patients, and children and adults with mental health problems in community day centres for special needs. These experiences helped me to develop strong leadership skills, compassion and excellent communication skills, as well as giving me the experience of working effectively within a team in a multi-disciplinary environment. This diversity of placements has provided me with a valuable understanding of the mental health and learning disability problems many individuals experience over the course of their life, and the importance of effective care and treatment to ensure the best quality of life possible.

As an active and sociable person outside work I enjoy walking, going to the gym, travelling the country with my family to support Cardiff City and visiting countries overseas I often accompany TOGS, a company run for able-bodied and disabled people, on visits to America and enjoy the social aspect and team spirit of such excursions. As well as being an experienced, mature person and a responsible parent, I believe I am a highly motivated individual, committed to achieving my goals. I am determined to fulfil my dream of a career in nursing and, although I know the course will be difficult, requiring stamina, hard work and self-discipline, I am looking forward to the challenges ahead. I hope to ultimately contribute to the field of nursing within the specialist area of learning disabilities and mental health and to practice my skills as a compassionate and dedicated nurse.

Example 14

In applying to study Nursing, I hope to pursue a rewarding job delivering primary patient care with the opportunity to constantly develop my knowledge.

Having decided on the need for a change of career, I am now working as a Nursing Assistant in a hospital, helping the staff with the personal care of patients, monitoring their condition, maintaining records and distributing medicines. This has given me an excellent insight into the running of a hospital and the reality of a nurse's working life. My job has taught me how to deal with potentially stressful and difficult situations, and to maintain a calm manner at all times. In particular, I have observed the importance of effective teamwork in ensuring the smooth running of a ward and the different contributions made by each member of the team. My first experience of care work was in helping to look after my mother during a terminal illness. As well as teaching me practical skills in handling and lifting, I have first hand experience of the effect such an illness can have on carers and loved ones and the need for a nurse to give empathy and support to patients' families. For me, the nurses were extremely useful in helping me to cope with our situation and I would like to offer the same service to other families during the most difficult periods of their lives.

In my previous employment, I have acquired a range of transferable skills which I will make use of as a student and during my career in nursing. As a Beauty Therapist I studied for NVQs which included particularly interesting sections on anatomy and physiology. My work involved daily interaction with customers, as well as responsibility for maintaining high levels of hygiene and cleanliness throughout the salon. I have also deputised for the manager on many occasions, taking full responsibility for the business in her absence. This has included dealing with unexpected situations, training new employees and controlling stock. My experience has developed in me strong interpersonal skills, with the ability to inform, instruct and advise people on all levels.

Since deciding on this change of career, I have been retaking my GCSEs in Maths and English, as they are a prerequisite of application, as well as taking Biology A level at a local college. This return to academic learning has been very enjoyable and has familiarised me with current educational practices. In my own time, I have been reading the BMJ online to improve my awareness of current issues in the medical profession and also subscribe to Nursing Standard which has been very informative. Combining these studies with my full time work has demanded very efficient time management skills and a strong commitment to the end goal.

Outside of work I enjoy attending the theatre and music concerts, as well as taking exercise outdoors such as bike rides and hill walks. I also enjoy the piano and have performed at several local music events and received several awards. In the long term I aim to become a Registered Nurse and then work my way up the nursing grades before specialising in a specific area. As a mature student who has given up a well-paid job to enter nursing, I am totally dedicated to practising as a nurse and I feel I have the skills and motivation necessary to succeed both during my training and in my future career.

Example 15

My desire to become a nurse began as a young child when I lived with and cared for my elderly grandmother who was severely disabled with arthritis. I loved being able to help her with the everyday tasks she was unable to fulfil on her own, not just out of a sense of duty and responsibility but also because it gave me a lot of pleasure and personal fulfilment to care for someone who needed help. From this time my ambition has always been to pursue a career in which I could work closely with people in a nurturing and caring environment, and where I could make a positive impact on both the lives of individuals and the community in which we live.

In order to realise my ambition to become a nurse I have maintained a disciplined and conscientious approach to my studies at school and college. I chose GCSE and A level subjects that would not only enable me to progress to university but also that stimulated my interest and broadened my outlook. I found the study of Sociology fascinating, particularly in the context of healthcare in our society and the perceived roles of the patient and the healthcare worker. Having researched further into this area of Sociology I have become very interested in the work of functional sociologist Talcott Parsons, whose social model of disability proposes that in defining disability in our society factors such as prejudice and exclusion, whether intended or not, play an important role. Also his theory that a sick person is not responsible for their condition and has a responsibility to seek help from the medical profession is one which is very thought-provoking and has encouraged me to look at the wider context of nursing. I believe as a healthy and able individual I have a social role to play in our society and am determined to apply my empathetic, caring nature to benefit others of all backgrounds and cultures.

There are many things that excite me about studying Nursing at university. Academically I am very keen to study the wide range of topics covered by the biological sciences, as well as the subjects offered in the Social Context of Health module, particularly Health Psychology, Sociology of Health and Illness, and Psychology, Gender and Health. My interest in Psychology was aroused during my A level course when I enjoyed examining some of the theories used to explain psychological issues surrounding certain behavioural traits within the context of cognitive and psychoanalysis. However, I am also looking forward to the challenges university life presents; meeting new people, studying and socialising together and offering support and friendship. I am aware that the Nursing course comprises both academic study and a strong practical element, and it is therefore important to understand the physical and emotional demands of nursing. With this in mind, and knowing the importance of relevant work experience prior to undertaking such a demanding career path, I have arranged for voluntary work experience at Dewsbury Hospital. During this placement I look forward to having the opportunity to shadow nurses and other healthcare workers as they perform a wide variety of tasks involving administration, hygiene procedures and patient contact.

In order to fulfil course assignments on schedule and maintain my own study programme I am able to prioritise tasks well and work efficiently with a disciplined and self-motivated approach. In this way, and by balancing the hard academic work with recreational and social pursuits such as badminton, netball, tennis and football, I believe I am well prepared for the challenges I will face. I consider myself to be a reliable, dedicated and enthusiastic person with an optimistic approach and a passion to succeed in my chosen vocation as a career nurse.

Example 16

In applying to study Nursing I hope to achieve my goal of working in one of the most emotionally satisfying professions available. With an ambition to specialise in mental health nursing, I look forward to providing a combination of mental well being and physical health to patients in my care. As a logical and practical individual I feel I am best suited to an approach to learning which combines academic and hands-on experience, such as that in Nursing.

My A level study of Physics and Maths has provided me with a logical approach to problem solving. I have learnt to apply a range of methods in order to find the most appropriate solution to problems with no obvious resolution and I have enjoyed adopting this logical thought process in everday situations. My skills in essay writing and analysis have been honed through English Literature and in studying a wide variety of texts, I have learnt to draw my own conclusions from a range of differing ideas and interpretations. I believe these skills in logical thought and analysis will help me in assessing the needs of patients and, subsequently, providing appropriate care. On top of my A level subjects I have undertaken an evening course in Counselling Skills and Psychology. This has instilled in me an open minded and non-judgemental approach to situations and individuals. I have also recently developed an interest in the portrayal of mental health in the media and have enjoyed reading Ken Kesey's 'One Flew Over the Cuckoo's Nest' and Susanna Kaysen's own memoirs of her time in a psychiatric hospital in 'Girl, Interrupted'. I believe the combination of my skills alongside my extra-curricular interests equip me well for a career in Mental Health Nursing.

A two-week work experience at a school for pupils with learning difficulties has furthered my desire to work in the caring profession. During my placement I was involved in organising a school production, helping to build scenery and make costumes and assisting the pupils in learning their lines. The rewards of seeing the production on opening night made the challenges faced in the preparation process more than worthwhile and gave me an overwhelming sense of pride. I was also able to observe how development is encouraged through creativity and how being involved in a group project allowed the children to develop socially.

In order to relax and maintain my own physical fitness, I practice yoga twice a week. I find this to be a very calming activity and it is one that I will continue at university in order to deal with the emotional and mental strain of a Nursing degree. For the past two years, I have also volunteered in a local charity shop, which has furthered my interpersonal skills and sense of responsibilitiy as well as allowing me to make a difference within the charity sector.

In conclusion, I have a firm understanding of the challenges that lie ahead for me at university and have ensured that I am well prepared to successfully take these on. I look forward to beginning my studies at your institution and fully immersing myself in university life.

Example 17

Having grown up in Malawi, an undeveloped country, I am keenly aware of the impact good health strategies and suitably informed policy makers can have on a country's health and social care system. My aim is to develop a fuller understanding of the factors affecting health, illness and recovery in the modern world and how they interact with each other. Having researched this course thoroughly I am confident that this area of study will offer me the opportunity to pursue a career dedicated to making a positive contribution to society.

Health is an issue that affects us all as individuals, families and members of local and global communities. Losing my mother to fungal meningitis and my father to HIV during my childhood, as well as other relatives due to the poor health strategies in my country, has given me a personal insight into the importance of this issue. It has also taught me that nothing in life comes easily, and I have taken responsibility for the wellbeing and financial security of my family since I was sixteen, giving me a mature and capable outlook. When my elder brother returned home to take over these responsibilities I began a new direction in life, coming to the UK and combining college study with my work as a healthcare assistant. Juggling these commitments has required time management, organisation and self motivation.

After working as a carer in a residential home, and at a variety of NHS hospitals via an agency, I became fascinated by the NHS system, and the people and policies that affect the way it is run. Through talking to my patients I have enjoyed learning about their conditions and treatments, their lifestyle, diet and general health patterns. As well as developing my curiosity about the healthcare sector, this has helped me to become a good listener and a confident communicator. In Malawi I was the head receptionist of a hotel, involving duties from welcoming guests and responding to complaints, to operating a large switchboard, preparing invoices and producing sales reports at the end of each day. I am currently working as a beauty consultant, advising people on how best to care for their skin, which has further improved my interpersonal skills.

My Health and Social Care course has been a useful introduction to the theory and practice of this sector and I have made use of the opportunity to refine my study skills to degree standard. At university I am looking forward to studying all aspects of the subject in detail, and particularly to examining health from a range of perspectives, from its biological bases to its political contexts.

In my leisure time I enjoy camping and travelling the UK sightseeing, learning new languages and socialising with people of different nationalities as well as keeping fit by working out, swimming and playing netball, for which I have won several trophies. I intend to continue these interests through clubs and societies at university. My long term career ambitions are to work in a management position within the NHS and I believe this course will equip me well for my desired progression. I am a highly motivated and ambitious student and I look forward to the challenges of university life.

Example 18

My motivation to study Nursing is my ambition to work in mental healthcare, using scientific knowledge and practical skills to assist mentally ill patients and their families through the most challenging times of their lives.

At school I have enjoyed learning about the systems of the human body, how they interact and how they can be kept healthy in Biology. My coursework investigating the components of a balanced diet was very interesting as I had to compare the quantities required of each food type, why they are needed, and the negative effects of not eating them. In Chemistry I enjoy conducting experiments and understanding which pieces of equipment are the most appropriate for each investigation. Studying Psychology has been fascinating and I feel this will be a useful basis for my degree level study as I have an appreciation of how the brain copes with stress and illness and have studied mental problems such as post-natal depression and how they can be prevented and treated. I look forward to building on this background at university and particularly to studying via practice-based learning as I feel this will be the best preparation for my future career. Having enjoyed working in groups during school coursework and presentations I am also looking forward to being part of a multidisciplinary medical team, integrating my expertise with that of social workers, psychiatrists and other heath and social care professionals.

For my Year 10 work experience I spent three weeks assisting in a nursing home for terminally ill patients. This was an eye-opening experience for me but I felt very inspired by the sensitivity and professionalism with which the nursing and care staff treated the patients and their families. My duties here involved washing and brushing patients' hair, making sure they were comfortable and chatting to them. I also made use of my previous experience of organising fundraising activities at school by arranging an evening of entertainment for the residents at the end of my stay. Working there was very rewarding as I could see the impact the extra personal attention could have on patients. Recently I spent a week shadowing a Community Nurse on her rounds, which included several visits to pregnant women. This increased my awareness of the different roles within the NHS and how they interact with each other, as well as the structure of the Trust system.

As a school House Prefect I work in a team with both staff and pupils to maintain discipline and a good atmosphere in the House, helping to develop my talents in organisation and communication. Adventure sports occupy much of my free time. I have several certificates in sailing, including night sailing and onboard emergency, and I go cross-country skiing as often as possible. I also enjoy cycling, squash and cross-country running and at university I intend to involve myself in organising events for clubs and societies. My travels have allowed me to be immersed in many different cultures and languages, giving me a more mature and humanitarian outlook. For my coming gap year I am planning to spend time in Canada training as a ski instructor, before returning home to work as a healthcare assistant. In the long term I hope to work as a successful Mental Health Nurse, adding to my skills by training throughout my career, and I look forward to taking full advantage of the opportunities available to me at university.

Example 19

Although I have harboured a lifelong ambition to qualify as a nurse, it was only recently that events in my personal life have inspired and motivated me to actively pursue this goal. My brother was diagnosed as diabetic last year and suffered convulsions while we were at a family meal; the feeling of helplessness due to not possessing the skills or knowledge to help him prompted me to reconsider my career path. Having also witnessed my grand mother deteriorating health caused by a stroke, and the aid that nurses have given both her and my brother on several occasions, it made me determined to gain a degree in Nursing so that I may help others in a similar fashion.

In returning to education, I strongly believe that I will benefit from a university course, especially as I experienced the methods of teaching involved while I was at college, e.g. lectures, followed by further private study and research. In order to supplement my knowledge I have joined St. John Ambulance and attend weekly meetings as well as events, which allow me to gain an insight into what life working in the healthcare profession would be like. It also enables me to gain a head start in terms of learning first aid, how to deal with emergencies, patient care and communication skills which will all form a vital part of my future studies and career.

I currently work for Inkjet Direct as a warehouse supervisor during the week and on Saturdays I attend the biggest computer show in England, selling to clients and individuals, giving advice and developing contacts. This latter role in particular has given me the confidence and ability to deal with people from all ethnicities and backgrounds. I have also had experience of working with children of all ages from volunteer work carried out at a local play-scheme and the school in which my mother teaches. I feel therefore that I am well equipped with the inter-personal skills which will be beneficial to me as a nurse.

As I will be starting the course as a 22-year-old I am confident that I will have the dedication and maturity to devote the majority of my time to my studies, especially as I have saved enough money to live on without having to hold down a job at the same time. I have already lived the 'student lifestyle' to a certain extent and so I understand the need for a healthy work/leisure balance. I live near the university so I will be able to visit the library and carry out further research in my free time, but I will also continue with my extra-curricular activities in order to relax and ease the pressure which a university degree inevitably brings. I am a keen runner and am currently training for the London marathon, having already completed several half-marathons. I also enjoy walks in the Lake District and participate in other sports such as paintballing and cycling. I fully intend to continue with these activities at university, hopefully joining the appropriate societies and clubs.

In concluding, I would like to reiterate that it has been my lifelong ambition to become a nurse. I have already made positive steps towards preparing myself for the degree and as a mature student I have that extra few years of experience which will help me to succeed. Studying Nursing at university will enable me to take the first step on the path to my ideal career, and I will make the most of the opportunities available to me.

Example 20

Since supporting my own mother through a terminal illness, and being highly impressed with the level of care and support we received as a family from the nurses and healthcare professionals, I have been interested in training in the area of nursing myself, in particular, I have an interest in working in the area of Adult Nursing. My first hand experience of coping with terminal illness will assist me in providing compassionate emotional support as well as practical advice. I feel confident I will be able to give patients and their families the support they need to get through such a traumatic time.

As a care assistant for a private medical group I visit patients of all ages in their homes to administer medicines, talking to them and providing emotional support. From this I have been able to learn about some common chronic health problems and their treatments. It has also shown me the importance of maintaining a calm professional and positive attitude towards patients, regardless of personal feelings. This is extremely important in a caring role, especially as many of my patients are terminally ill and have few visitors. I have found I have a particular talent for using my communication skills to help patients stay positive.

In order to prepare for attending university I have been completing a two year part-time Access to Healthcare course. Studying the sociological aspects of nursing has been particularly fascinating, allowing me to understand the range of outside factors which may affect a person's health and response to treatment. I have also made the most of the opportunity to familiarise myself with writing essays, taking exams and remembering and applying information. As part of my course I spent a week shadowing a hospital nurse, learning about a typical day and the practical requirements, such as energy and stamina, required. This has confirmed my desire to become a nurse and I will be undertaking a further work placement with a Community Nurse next month. During my degree I am very excited about the opportunity to implement the theories we will learn on the hospital wards during block placements. I am also looking forward to studying the medical aspects of the degree.

In my leisure time I enjoy keeping fit through running and other outdoor activities. I also enjoy travelling around Britain and visiting sites of historic interest, particularly early Tudor architecture. Raising my family, and combining this with studying and full-time employment, has tested my organisational skills such as management, budgeting, childcare and first aid. As a mature applicant I have had to make many changes to my family life in order to make it possible to return to education and I am fully committed to achieving my goal of training and practising as a nurse.

Example 21

Nursing has always appealed to me as a career through which I can utilise my interpersonal skills and empathetic nature to help others to improve their quality of life. A lack of confidence initially held me back from focusing on my own development and pursuing this career. However, after observing friends and acquaintances benefit from returning to education and realising their ambitions, and having raised my family to school age, I now feel in a position to commit myself fully to returning to university and studying Nursing.

Volunteering once a week for several years at a drop-in centre for women with addictions has given me valuable experience of providing non-judgemental support and advice. The women who use the centre are usually dependent on drugs or alcohol and many are prostitutes and homeless. Working with them has given me a taste of some of the difficult situations a healthcare professional may be involved in and has demonstrated the need for clear, sensitive and effective communication skills and a combination of empathy and emotional resilience. As I am sometimes left in charge at the centre I have also developed strengths in leadership, organisation and management. Since February 2008 I have also spent every Friday evening hosting a youth club attended by around forty teenagers, which has developed my ability to communicate with young people and my understanding of some of the difficulties they may face. Combined with previous employment experience as a nanny in London and abroad, this has ensured that I have an affinity for young children and experience of a care-giving role.

My career has equipped me with a range of relevant skills. After being a full-time nanny for seven years, making the most of the opportunity to travel around the world meeting new people and exploring new cultures, I worked as an accounts assistant to a catering firm. This involved liaising with staff and customers and performing all aspects of the company's accounts, requiring proficient numerical and administrative skills as well as an appreciation of teamwork. As a financial assistant, I later handled large sums of money via a computerised system, developing my IT skills and initiative and familiarising myself with the importance of discretion and confidentiality. As I also had a supervisory role on occasion, I became adept at leading and organising others. I have also worked in a call centre, utilising my interpersonal skills to reassure customers who had broken down and liaising with breakdown mechanics to arrange recovery.

At present I am studying an Access course, which has provided me with an excellent reintroduction to studying and ensured I am proficient in writing essays, conducting research and delivering presentations. I have thoroughly enjoyed having the opportunity to follow up issues of academic interest to me and discuss them in class. I look forward to continuing this at university, learning from the experience and opinions of others as well as sharing my own. In particular I am keen to study the aspects of Sociology and Psychology that support much of the theory of Nursing.

As a mature applicant I have researched my career options thoroughly and I am confident that I have the personality and qualities to become a successful nurse. I look forward to tackling the challenges of degree level study and am committed to experiencing all that university life has to offer.

Example 22

As a future nurse I look forward to working as part of a multi-disciplinary team of health professionals providing care and support to vulnerable members of society. Having witnessed a close relative suffer from autism, and the help they have received from social workers and nurses alike, has inspired me to specialise in the area of Learning Disability Nursing. Studying Sociology A level as well as Sciences, the sociological factors involved in general well-being are of particular interest to me. As such, I am looking forward to furthering my understanding of this area at university, focusing on issues facing individuals with learning difficulties and how best to support them as they develop social relationships and networks.

Whilst completing my A levels part-time I have also been working as a volunteer support worker. This role involves providing care and support to individuals with disabilities in a residential setting, doing their shopping, helping to prepare meals and keeping their living environment clean and tidy. Above all, the most rewarding aspect of the role is in befriending the residents, spending time listening and talking with them. This has instilled in me a sensitivity to people's needs and the ability to form relationships with clients and their families in providing individualised care. Furthermore, it has provided me with the compassion and communication skills required of a nurse and has confirmed my desire to work within Learning Disability Nursing. I look forward to enhancing these skills through placement opportunities during my degree.

Through taking a gap year I hope to broaden my experience of different cultures and languages, and will be funding my own travels. Using my organisational and planning abilities I have arranged a round the world trip which will include three months volunteering at a

Red Cross orphanage in Japan and one month teaching at a school in Kenya. I will be working full-time as a support worker until March and on returning from my travels, I will be volunteering as a carer in the UK with CSV. As well as being an exciting experience I hope it will help to improve my confidence, interpersonal skills and independence during my year out, which will be useful on starting at university.

At school I enjoy playing on the basketball, rugby and chess teams. Using my leadership skills I also set up and now manage a basketball club for Lower School children. As part of my school's volunteering programme I have spent three months mentoring primary school children in English and Maths. This has been a rewarding way to contribute to the community and has taught me valuable communicative and interpersonal techniques. I also enjoy taking part in extreme sports such as wakeboarding and surfing whenever I can. As a highly motivated and well-rounded individual I intend to make a positive contribution to university life and look forward to facing the challenges of higher education.

Example 23

Finding my present career unfulfilling, and having experienced a variety of caring and childcare roles, I am now hoping to qualify as a nurse. This has been my ambition for many years and as my children are now older, and I have completed college courses in preparation for tertiary level study, I feel I am now able to commit myself fully to this major career change.

Re-entering the academic world has been an exciting experience for me and I am eager to learn more. Through studying for my BTEC First Diploma in Caring I have encountered a variety of aspects of healthcare. This knowledge added an extra dimension to my employment as a Personal Care Assistant. Caring for an MS sufferer I have had an insight into daily life in a healthcare role. I use an overhead hoist, slide sheets, and shower and toileting chairs as part of his daily routine, as well as preparing his food, and preparing his medication under his supervision. I developed effective communication skills and an empathetic approach, respecting the man's wishes and ensuring his safety at all times. Motivating and supporting him emotionally was important, and I implemented aspects of my college work such as understanding others' needs, and sensitivity to personal preferences.

Currently I am about to start a new Healthcare Assistant job, working on a Rehab and Therapies ward for people with neurological conditions. Here I will gain experience of working in a busy hospital, assisting with feeding, toileting and bathing, and maintaining the relevant paperwork. I aim to make full use of this opportunity to learn from others working in a variety of medical roles on the ward.

In my career as a Catering Manager I acquired skills and experiences which I can bring to my degree studies as well as future nursing work. Catering for a secondary school of 1,000 pupils I managed eight members of staff. This involved preparing rota menus, monitoring stock, maintaining accounts and written records, following company and Health and Safety guidelines, and training staff to do the same. Providing supportive leadership, I became experienced in managing limited time and resources efficiently, using my initiative to solve problems as they arose, and prioritising and delegating tasks effectively. Liaising with a variety of staff, children, and a range of educational professionals, I am adept at listening and communicating to people on all levels and respecting the diversity of our community. I have had a successful career, which I combined with raising my family, and I will bring the same hardworking, hands-on approach to nursing.

Outside of my family and professional life I work out at the gym when time allows and I have just taken up golf. I also enjoy horse-riding, having owned my own horse in the past, as well as cooking and spending time with my family.

In the long term I aim to practise as a qualified Midwife or Paediatric Nurse. Having personal experience of complications in pregnancy as well as raising my own children, I am particularly keen to contribute to patient care in this field. As a mature student undergoing a complete career change I have researched my options very carefully. I am a strong willed and highly motivated person, dedicated to becoming a nurse, and I feel I have the skills and commitment required to achieve my ambition.

Example 24

My motivation to study Nursing stems from my desire to embark on a career that is both challenging and rewarding, and one that will allow me to make a valid contribution to people's lives. I perceive nursing as a profession for dedicated and reliable people who are able to build relationships quickly. These are qualities which I posses and I genuinely believe I can contribute greatly to the world of nursing.

Through my A level studies I have developed an organised and systematic approach to managing my workload, a skill I feel is essential in undertaking degree level study. I have greatly enjoyed the subjects of Psychology and Sociology as both have given me the opportunity to improve my understanding of human interactions. Sociology in particular furthered my interest in this field through studying the interactions of vulnerable individuals with the wider community and the reasons why some people struggle to integrate into society. I look forward to expanding my knowledge in this area and the ways in which nurses can aid in the integration process. I especially enjoy applying theory to practical settings and look forward to combining my academic study with clinical placements.

Outside of my academic achievements, I am involved in the Duke of Edinburgh scheme and have achieved my bronze and silver level awards. Working as part of a group to complete tasks within the scheme has enabled me to become an effective team player, a skill I believe will be useful in my career as I will use this strength to successfully communicate with other healthcare professionals in order to provide the highest standards of patient care. I am also involved in providing learning support to a Year 8 pupil with additional needs, helping her with daily activities such as note taking and personal time management, as well as helping her to overcome the challenges faced in living with learning difficulties. I find this very rewarding as I can see the impact my assistance has on her life and it has demonstrated the importance of patience and a willingness to listen in providing effective care.

My work experiences have provided me with further insight into the world of the caring professions. Through school I took part in a placement at a day care centre which involved providing support to elderly people and their carers. This was an eye-opening experience as it showed me that the role goes much further than providing patient care, but also to caring for their friends and families. Following on from my enjoyment of this, I arranged my own work placement at a local hospital. This gave a contrasting view of healthcare and allowed me to observe what working in a hospital setting would be like. Both experiences have encouraged me to pursue a career in nursing and prior to commencing my studies, I plan to work as a nursing auxiliary through the nurse bank.

In the future I would like to specialise in Learning Disability Nursing and I see my studies as the first step towards a career I am passionate about. As the role of the nurse becomes more involved with patient welfare, so too does the job become more demanding. I believe I have the skills and qualities required to meet these demands and look forward to taking advantage of the opportunities available to me, both as a student and a future nurse.

Chapter 3

Example 25

My motivation to study Nursing at university is my desire to combine an academic interest in health science with my intention to pursue a career as a qualified professional within the NHS. My fourteen years of employment experience within healthcare have given me a sound understanding of the NHS health and care systems and of the different professional roles within them. Having previously begun a degree course in Nursing, which was cut short when I was forced to leave university for personal reasons, I have a realistic impression of what my degree studies will involve. Although having to abandon my previous degree course was a significant setback, it has not affected my enthusiasm for the subject and I am now more committed than ever to achieving my ambition.

Working as a support worker and carer, helping people with various physical and mental disabilities and health problems to remain in their own home, has given me valuable experience of delivering practical care to patients. It has also ensured that I have the skills in communication, adaptability, stamina, team working and initiative which are required for a career in healthcare. I am familiar with adopting a holistic approach to patient care and am proficient in following care plans, reporting changes, dealing sensitively with patients' families and being aware of my professional limitations. As a healthcare assistant, I was a member of a multidisciplinary team and dealt with patients, carers and medical and nursing staff on a daily basis, giving me confidence in my interpersonal abilities and an insight into the running of a hospital. Further to this, I also have experience of working as a carer in a mental health hospital for the elderly and have also observed qualified nurses working in both NHS and private settings. I have made the most of these opportunities to learn as much as possible about the career paths and training available within this field. At university I am looking forward to building on my previous experience during the practical placements in different settings and to developing the skills to evaluate, restore and maintain the physical functions of the body alongside providing care and support to patients from all walks of life, their families and carers.

As part of my commitment to my professional development I am currently studying for an NVQ in Health and Social Care and a Level 4 Diploma in Caring for People with Learning Disabilities. Both of these courses are distance learning, requiring me to be disciplined and self-motivated and to manage my time effectively. I have very much enjoyed my continued involvement in education and I am looking forward to embarking on full-time study. In my spare time I enjoy keeping fit through swimming and wall climbing and I also enjoy travelling and exploring new regions. One day I hope to have the opportunity to diversify my professional experience by spending some time working in developing countries.

As a mature student embarking on a career change I have invested a great deal in my return to full-time education and I have investigated my career options fully. My employment experience and previous study of Healthcare has confirmed my choice of a new career direction. After graduation I intend to work as a qualified nurse within the NHS and I am confident that this degree program will equip me with the skills and expertise to achieve this goal.

Chapter 8

Proofreading your Personal Statement

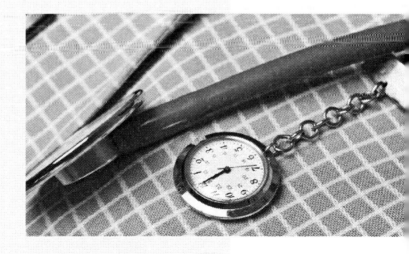

Proofreading your Personal Statement

When you believe that you are ready to submit your Personal Statement, **don't** until you are sure you are happy with its final format. It is also very useful to ask other people to read through your final version; it is amazing how helpful it is to obtain the viewpoint from 'a fresh pair of eyes'. For example, it may be very useful to receive the comments from an English teacher, especially with regard to your punctuation and writing style. Equally, there may be people you met during your work experience who would be pleased to help you in this way. **However**, remember that it is **your** Personal Statement and if you feel passionate about an issue to the point that you are determined to include it, then do so!

Final checklist:

- Do you have a punchy and attention grabbing introduction?
- Do you come over as passionate about studying Nursing?
- Do you indicate that you have given serious practical consideration to the implications of establishing a nursing career for **you**?
- Do you describe how your academic and extra-curricular activities have helped you to make this choice?
- Is every piece of information you provide clearly relevant to your application to study Nursing?
- Is your Personal Statement arranged in paragraphs? Is it balanced? Does it flow?
- Does your Personal Statement contain a concluding paragraph?
- Check all spelling and all punctuation.

Submitting your application

The majority of applications to study Nursing are submitted electronically. Your Personal Statement needs to be typed up electronically and must not exceed 47 lines and 4,000 characters (~580–620 words, size 12 Times New Roman).

If you are applying through your school or college, you will be provided with directions as to how to proceed. Those applying independently, such as graduates or mature students, can register directly on the UCAS website.

For more information visit www.ucas.com

Key points

Keep looking for ways to improve upon your draft effort.

Invite others to proofread your statement before you finally submit it.

Chapter 9

Things to avoid

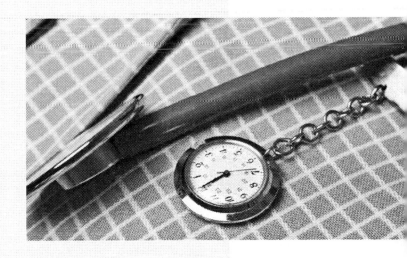

Things to avoid

This guide has focused upon helping you how to draft, structure, refine and proofread your Personal Statement.

Here is a list of some things to avoid!

- Rushing the preparation of your Personal Statement – you will need plenty of time to write it!
- Needlessly repeating information that is contained in other parts of your application.
- Relying on a spell checking function – check it yourself; use a dictionary.
- Dishonesty, or deliberately misleading the reader.
- Using any word or phrase the meaning of which you are uncertain.
- Trying to be funny. Just play it straight.
- Drawing attention to any weakness, unless you have learnt from it, handled it, and become a more complete person.
- Including comments which criticise others or casting yourself in a favourable light in comparison to others.
- Simply listing achievements or interests; every comment must be relevant. Lists make for dry reading!
- Disjointed statements. Readers do not like having to flick backwards and forwards when trying to understand your comments.
- Overuse of the 'I' word.
- Lack of structure; lack of paragraphs.
- Not proofreading your statement – ask your teachers, friends and family to help you in this regard. But remember that it is **your** Personal Statement!

Key points

First, always make sure that your Personal Statement really is unique to you.

Second, make sure you keep a copy. You can be sure that if you are called for interview, panel members are almost certain to question you specifically upon some of the comments you have made. For you to say 'Oh, I forgot I wrote that' would give an incredibly bleak impression!

Chapter 10

Information for teachers and parents

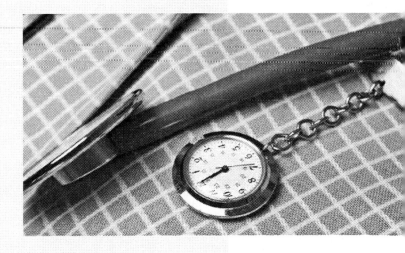

Chapter 10

Information for teachers and parents

In a sense, the hardest aspect of writing a Personal Statement is staring at a blank piece of paper and actually beginning the process. The best way to help someone who is struggling to get to grips with their Personal Statement is to talk through their academic and personal achievements with them, and encourage them to think about the skills and personality traits they have developed and which they are particularly proud of. If a young person is finding it difficult to be enthusiastic about the prospect of writing a university Personal Statement, first encourage them to enthuse about their hobbies and pastimes in open discussion, and use this as a springboard to launching into the 'thought showering' process.

Possible areas to discuss with an applicant include:

*   Topics they have particularly enjoyed learning about whilst studying for their A levels. Why did they enjoy this area – what skills did it allow them to demonstrate and develop? (i.e. a History project enabled them to discover their enjoyment of researching in a library, or studying 'group theory' in Psychology has given them new insights into their relationships at school).
*   Career aims – where do they see themselves in ten years' time? What personal traits and attributes do they think will help them succeed?
*   What achievements, both in and out of school, are they particularly proud of? How has participating in these activities developed them as a person?

Once a young person has drafted their first attempt at their Personal Statement, you can help them further by proofreading it and offering constructive criticism. In addition, consider their first draft in the light of the following checklist:

- Does it contain a punchy and relatively attention grabbing introduction?
- Does it explain their reasons for choosing to study Nursing?
- Does it state what they are looking forward to learning more about?
- Does it state their future career goals?
- Does it state how their academic and extracurricular activities have developed them as an individual?
- Is the information included relevant to their course choice?
- Is the Personal Statement arranged in paragraphs?
- Does the Personal Statement contain a short concluding paragraph?

Chapter 11

Closing thoughts

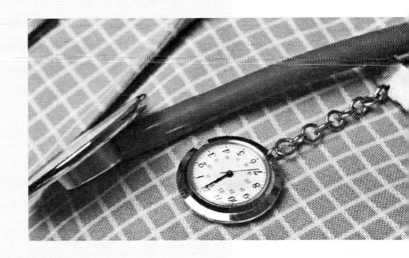

Closing thoughts

The aim of this guide is to provide you with a good idea of what should be included in your Personal Statement for application to study Nursing in the UK. Our hope is that by following the principles and steps contained in this guide you will be able to compose a well-structured and effective Personal Statement.

For more information on how BPP Learning Media can support you with your application to university please visit:

www.bpp.com/health

We strongly recommend that you do seek more information from university websites, and advice from staff at the universities you wish to attend, to ensure that your Personal Statement contains the information that they request.

From all of us at BPP Learning Media we would like to wish you every success in securing your place at university.

Good Luck!!

Appendix
Useful websites

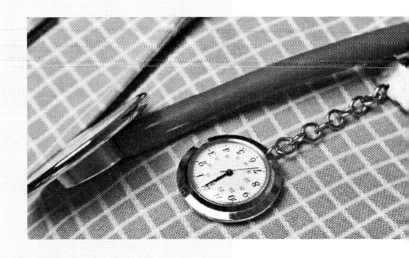

Appendix

Useful websites

Universities and Colleges Admissions Service
www.ucas.com

Nursing and Midwifery Council
www.nmc-uk.org

Royal College of Nursing
www.rcn.org.uk

NHS Careers
www.nhscareers.nhs.uk

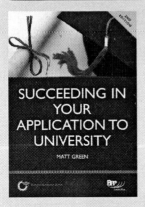
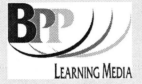

More titles in the Entry to University Series

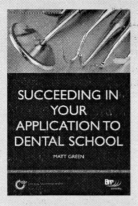

SUCCEEDING IN YOUR APPLICATION TO DENTAL SCHOOL

MATT GREEN

As the competition for Dental School places continues to increase, it is more important than ever to ensure that your application reflects what the admissions tutors will be looking for. This book will help school leavers, graduates and mature individuals applying to Dental School, together with parents and teachers, to make their UCAS Personal Statement both compelling and convincing reading. In this book, Matt Green:

- Describes the context of the Dental School Personal Statement within the application process

- Highlights the fact that selection for Dental School implies selection for the dental profession

- Sets out the essential contents of the Dental Personal Statement, the key steps in its preparation, what to include and what not to include

- Drafts and refines a fictitious UCAS Personal Statement, making for a most valuable case study through which the consideration of all the key principles are brought to life

- Includes 30 high quality Personal Statement examples to provide inspiration during the writing process

Sep 2011
Paperback
978-1-445379-63-0

By using this engaging, easy to use and comprehensive book, you can remove so much of the uncertainty surrounding your Dental School application.

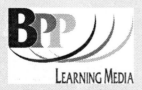

LEARNING MEDIA

More titles in the Entry to Medical School Series

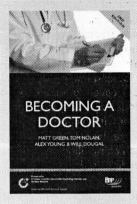

Deciding on whether or not to pursue a career in medicine is a decision that should not be taken lightly. Becoming a doctor can be highly rewarding but is not without its drawbacks. It is therefore important that you gain a clear insight into the world of medicine to ensure that it is the right path for you to follow.

This book has been written with the above in mind to provide a clear picture of what becoming a doctor really involves. In this comprehensive book Matt Green and Tom Nolan explore:

October 2011

Paperback

978-1-445381-51-0

- What it really means to be a good doctor

- The steps that should be taken to confirm whether a career in medicine is really the one for you

- How to successfully apply to medical school including the various entrance exams (UKCAT, BMAT, GAMSAT), the UCAS personal statement and subsequent medical school interview

- Life as a student at medical school and how to excel

- The various career paths open to you as a doctor with invaluable insights provided by practising doctors.

This engaging and comprehensive book is essential reading for anyone serious about becoming a doctor and determining whether it really is the right career for you!

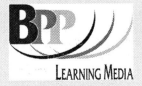

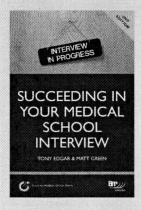
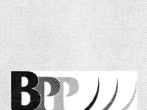